Herbalism For Beginners:
The Complete Guide To Herbal Remedies And How You Can Grow Them At Home

The Power Of Alternative Medicine

By Jolanny Lopez

Herbalism For Beginners: The Complete Guide To Herbal Remedies And How You Can Grow Them At Home
Copyright © 2020 by Jolanny Lopez

For information contact :
jolannylopez@gmail.com

First Edition: June 2020

Table Of Contents

Introduction

Due to many factors that cannot be helped, including age and stress, the human body undergoes natural wear and tear as we progress with our daily activities. Apart from natural damage, several bacteria can attack the body to the point that it needs restoration. The process of healing the human body has surely undergone major changes over thousands of years. Old cultures like the Romans, Greeks, Chinese, Egyptians, and Indians practiced holistic medicine for centuries. Technological advancements have dragged the medical world into an obsessive dependence on drugs, supplements, and endless procedures. The economic gains that drive today's medicine have made light of the extreme value of the practice and snuffed out the original essence of healing and wellness. This has greatly obscured the healing process, making many of us wonder if we should be running back to methods of old for wholeness, healing, and well-being.

Alternative Medicine: Herbalism Over Traditional Medicine

Today, alternative medicine, the complementary, integrative, and holistic treatments used simultaneously with or in place of traditional treatment, is making a comeback and gaining international acceptance. Herbalism is one of the most popular alternative therapies available in our modern-day. Herbalism employs the use of natural remedies to treat and prevent illnesses as well as nurture good health. The use of plants and herbs for their therapeutic qualities is not a new concept, the practice is almost as old as time itself. Modern synthetic application of this method has been in an upward trend for years in the West. Herbalists recommend particular herbs to be used alone or in conjunction with other ingredients for the treatment of varied ailments. Because of their pure form, these herbal remedies are scarcely followed by the adverse side effects associated with modern-day pharmaceuticals.

There is an increasing body of evidence to substantiate alternative medical recommendations like herbalism. One study carried out in Germany showed that dissatisfaction with conventional medical treatment was one of the leading reasons why people preferred herbalism as a method of treatment over traditional methods. Even big medical centers like Yale, Stanford, and Harvard have welcomed integrative medicine. Although people are aware of the limitations of herbal medicine and hardly turn to them for acute cases, they would rather turn to herbalism than go to the hospital with an illness. People use herbal medicine to handle mild to moderate illnesses or start treating their illnesses with herbal remedies before going to the hospital to report advanced cases. They wouldn't keep trusting herbalism unless they are seeing notable benefits.

What Will you Gain from Herbal Medicine

The way of herbal medicine seeks to place the body in a state of natural balance so that it heals itself. Different herbs are used as active ingredients to treat different ailments. Some common medicinal herbs and their benefits include:

- Echinacea helps to fight infections and boosts the immune system.
- Ginseng aids recovery from sickness by treating fatigue.
- Dong Quai is used to treat gynecological ailments, period pain, and menopause.

Modern medicine is established upon herbal remedies. Herbal remedies boast of many benefits with significantly lower side effects than traditional drugs. Why then is herbal medicine not taking center stage in health and wellness? Here are some more reasons why you should be using medicinal herbs to boost your immune system. Herbal medicine is:

- Easier to get than prescriptions.
- More pocket friendly than traditional medicine.
- Possesses strong natural healing properties.
- Strengthens the human immune system.

Herbal Medicine Works

Every year, an estimated 35 billion dollars is spent on alternative medicine in the United States. Around 40% of the American population have tried at least one form of alternative medicine at one time. These figures only go to show the seriousness of the industry and how many people are jumping in to enjoy the benefits. While herbalists extract active ingredients from whole parts of plants, some pharmaceutical drugs are still manufactured using one part of a plant as the active ingredient. The result is that the impact of these pharmaceutical drugs is lessened. For example, the salicylic acid used in the manufacture of aspirin is derived from meadowsweet. Aspirin can cause bleeding in the stomach lining but organic meadowsweet includes other compounds to stop irritation from salicylic acid.

Many people are reaping the serious benefits of using medicinal herbs in their life. Heidi Villegas, a mum, and blogger is a shining example. Heidi records in her blog that herbalism for her is an art and learning how to use herbs has transformed her life for good. She states that she lived the modern life of convenience going from doctor to drugstore whenever she got sick until she started reading and learning about herbs. She had to research everything she knows and is now passionate about sharing her knowledge with the world so others can enjoy the full benefits of ancient herbal remedies too.

I promise you that herbal medicine works and using information from this book, and other exhaustive resources will put you on a new health path you will never end up regretting. Herbal remedies have been useful for thousands of years, they are good now and they will always be advantageous to all-round wholeness.

What Are you Waiting for?

Making use of ancient recipes and extracting the whole benefits of herbs is easy and doesn't constitute a huge lifestyle change. This book contains everything you need to know about herbs to get you started on your journey to enjoying the best herbal remedies. Loaded with the knowledge you will get from this in-depth resource, you can begin using herbs in homemade remedies that will boost your immune system and that of your family members. Don't wait another day, week, or year to jump into this highly beneficial sea of healthiness. Most medicinal herbs carry loads of healing compounds in one package. It is better to consume them whole as tinctures and teas than as a single compound worked on through laboratory processes. Always make sure you're using the right plant and taking the right parts of that plant and remember that cooked herbs keep all their benefits.

Chapter One
The History of Herbalism

When faced with ailments and health issues, the human race has had to come up with ways of keeping themselves healthy and thriving. From the beginning of time, viruses, infections, injuries, and illnesses have been and still are the biggest enemy of mankind.

In the search for answers, our ancestors have come across plants. They started watching their animals eat them and wondered whether or not it was worth investigating and using them to heal their sick ones.

In this chapter, we will be looking at Herbal medicine throughout history, from the first historical records of humanity's findings to the modern-day herbalists who benefit from said findings and continue to add new information to the list through the science we call Botany. To create an informed and realistic view on what herbalism is and its benefits, we need to pay attention to the past and what it teaches us about the way people saw it for thousands of years and how their view changed through the centuries.

Herbalism has its roots deep in antiquity, predating written human history. And as we can't be certain of how it all started we can assume that women were the ones to first practice it.

In the early ancient times, men were the hunters and women the gatherers. They would use everything they would find in nature to cook, make clothing, and heal ailments. We can assume that to figure out what is poisonous and what is safe they had to look at animals and communicate with other women about their findings. If someone would have gotten poisoned, they would know which plant to avoid. As this is only speculation because there is no written evidence of this being true, many scientists believe it to be very probable giving the way ancient families had to divide labor.

The first written record of plants used for a medicinal purpose was created over five thousand years ago by the Sumerians, on clay tablets in modern Iraq or the ancient Mesopotamia. They created lists of hundreds of medicinal plants such as opium and myrrh. The writings show us today the importance of plants to our ancient ancestors. They considered their discoveries worth writing down even though, writing in those times was scarce and difficult. It shows us the kind of respect the Sumerians had for plants and their potential benefits.

A few millenniums later, around the year 1500BCE, the Ancient Egyptians wrote a document known as the "Papyrus Ebers" listing over 850 herbal medicines we recognize and use today.

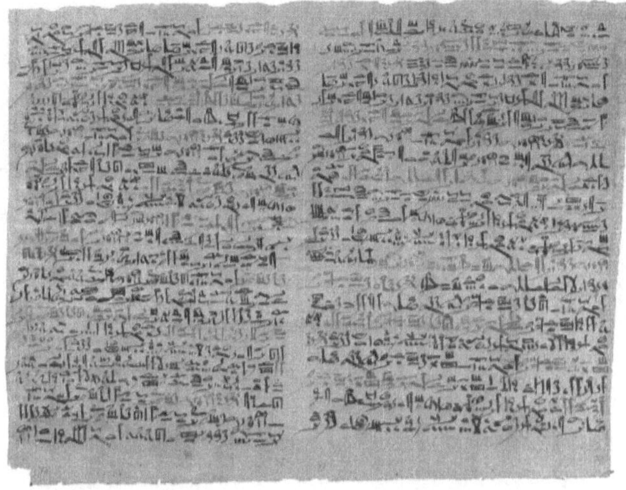

The Papyrus lists ailments and treatments from "disease of the limbs" to "disease of the skin". Some of the plants listed as treatments were garlic, juniper, cannabis, castor bean, aloe, and mandrake. In the way they were writing, the symptoms seemed to be regarded as the disease itself and the treatments were aimed at treating the symptoms. Scientists do not doubt that the Papyrus document was carried around the world through trade and politics, influencing and evolving the way many cultures perceived medicine. Some tomb illustrations and jars containing traces of herbs also serve as evidence for these findings.

Looking at ancient Egyptians today we can be certain they possessed great knowledge in various subjects as they used to write down on stone everything they deemed important and we can read and translate today the hieroglyphs to learn from their cultures. The Papyrus writings seemed to be of great importance to them, as they made sure to preserve it very carefully. Most of their knowledge of medicine and illnesses were being registered in these ancient books. The respect they had for plants is undeniable and their discoveries on their usefulness regarding symptoms seem to be undeniable.

In India, around 4000 BC Sanskrit writings such as the Rig Veda and Atharva Veda were some of the earliest writings that formed the basis of the Ayurveda system, one of the oldest healing systems. It was based on the belief that health and wellness depend on the balance between the body, mind, and spirit. This system used turmeric along with many other herbs and minerals described by ancient Indian herbalists like Charaka and Sushruta during the year 1000 BC. Indians seemed to have been the first ones who understood the importance of plants in healing, so far so they built a whole healing system around it.

In ancient China, a mythological Chinese emperor named Shennong is said to have written the first Chinese pharmacopeia, the "Shennong Ben Cao Jing", listing 365 medicinal plants and their uses, including Ephedra, a shrub used to introduce ephedrine to modern medicine, hemp and chaulmoogra, one of the first effective treatments for leprosy.

From ancient times, the Chinese have kept their herbalist traditions, being the biggest herbalist community in the world in our modern times. They still practice herbal medicine and use remedies they've known to work for centuries. They use herbalism in conjunction with Western medicine and they protect their bodies using plants before they even get. So instead of going to the doctors after illnesses already affect their bodies and health, they go to the doctors more often and use plant-based remedies and treatments to strengthen their bodies and protect them from possible illnesses and diseases. We should pay attention to eastern medicine and their practices because they must have kept their traditions for a reason.

One of the famous if not the most famous physicians of all time is Hippocrates. He lived between 460-377 BC in Greece and believed that our bodies became diseased naturally and the diseases were not caused by superstitions or by God, unlike the popular belief in those days. While in prison for holding opposing views to the authorities of his days, he wrote the book "The Complicated Body" which consisted of many medical theories considered true today, and he is often referred to as the "Father of Modern Medicine ". The Hippocratic Oath is being taken by the ones who complete medical degrees in our modern days. He used many herbal medicines and said the famous words"let your foods be your medicines, and your medicines your foods". He wrote about the willow bark and its properties, giving the information scientists needed to synthesize the active compounds of willow to make aspirin.

The Hippocratic Corpus was composed of many writing and books that are associated with Hippocrates and his findings, it was written by both Hippocrates and the ones who followed and respected his way of perceiving medicine. Though many of the plants mentioned in The Hippocratic Corpus were similar to those used by religious sectors of healing, they differ in the reasoning behind using them. That being logical and experimental, much like Hippocrates used to think. He intended to give plants the scientific-based recognition using his practical and natural way of seeing medicine. Western medicine itself was based on plants and scientists today are in the process of proving the great effects plants have on the human body.

We will continue to look at ancient Greece and Rome and the people who made remarkable discoveries in herbal medicine.

Galen of Pergamon, a Greek physician practicing in Rome wrote many books on the medicinal use of plants with one of the most notable being "Works of Therapeutics". In this book, he was discussing the connection between many disciplines and medicine and how they can work together to restore people's health and well-being. He also played a very important role in Humoralism, a system of medicine created to detail the make-up and the workings of the human body. His role in this system was important for how pharmacists learned to organize their remedies after understanding how each human body is different.

Diocles of Carystus was a Greek physician and writer who lived close to Hippocrates' times. He was referred to as the second Hippocrates because of his comprehensive work and similarity to Hippocrates' views. He is thought to have written the first medical book tough the evidence for this has been lost. However, his work was mentioned in many modern scientists' writings as well as his contemporaries' gaining enough respect to have his advice on herbal medicine taken seriously.

Pliny the Elder was a Roman author, naturalist, and natural philosopher. He wrote the book "Natural History" as a comprehensive guide to nature, presenting an extensive catalog of herbs valuable to medicine. This catalog with over 900 listed drugs and plants, brings great value to our current knowledge of herbal medicine, standing at the base of what we understand about nature and its healing abilities.

Pedanius Dioscorides, stepping on Pliny's steps, a great physician himself, wrote another pharmacopeia called "De Materia Medica" which means "Of medical matters". The books consist of over 1000 medicines produced from herbs, minerals, and animals. The remedies in the pharmacopeia were widely used through ancient times, making Dioscorides an expert on drugs for almost two millenniums after his death.

Theophrastus' book "Historia Plantarum" is also worth mentioning in the history of herbalism as it was the first systematization of the botanical world. These Greek and Roman philosophers and scientists were the ones who spread Herbalism and the knowledge they gathered throughout the whole world. We will look at how their discoveries impacted medicine for the many years to come starting in the Middle Ages.

Through the Middle Ages, the monasteries in Britain and mainland Europe started preserving herbalism. Monasteries were serving as medical schools before the establishment of universities in the 11th and 12th centuries. Monks were transcribing and copying the works of Galen, Dioscorides, and Hippocrates while growing the most common and useful herbs in their "Physick" gardens to teach the next generation of monks and future physicians.

The nun monasteries were also trying to spread the knowledge of the ancient physicians on plants as remedies for illnesses. We can assume the reason monasteries took over as places of healing for people could have been based on their religious beliefs as plants were used in antiquities by pagans and witches. There is evidence that the Christian Church has attempted through history to take over the practices of pagans and witches and give them to God in a new and less superstitious way.

In the 6th and 7th centuries, after the Islamic conquest of North Africa, many eastern scholars have acquired the medical writings of the Greeks and Romans. Avicenna, an Iranian physician, combined the writings of Galen and Dioscorides on herbal medicine with the ones of his own people and wrote "The Cannon of Medicine". The Cannon of Avicenna spread through Europe in the 11th and 12th centuries and is considered one of the most influential texts ever written. The History of Medicine makes an important reference to Avicenna's work as the basis for medicine and herbalism in particular.

After the invention of the printing press in the mid 15th century, the herbal remedies of Dioscorides, Galen and Avicenna started to be mass-produced and sold outside the palaces, monasteries, and universities. The use of the herbal medicines didn't require special skills, the readers would gather the herbs and apply them as prescribed.

In those times there were many writers who were looking to revolutionize medicine and find new plant-based remedies. One of the most famous ones was Paracelsus (1493-1541). He emphasized the patient experience and how ignorant it would have been to follow blindly the ancient physicians.

Even though he made very clear his distrust in traditional herbalism, Paracelsus brought back to life the 1st-century "doctrine of signatures" which stated that every plant has its specific sign. It explains how the color, shape, appearance, and environment of a plant indicates it's medicinal use. For example, the pansies with their heart-shaped petals were used for heart problems. This doctrine of signatures was recognized by the physicians of those days and started gaining popularity in the western world.

Englishman, Nicholas Culpeper, a century later, revived another ancient part of herbalism: astrology. In astrological herbalism, herbs were connected to zodiac signs. They treated illnesses by looking at the part of the body affected and finding the sign or planet that ruled over it. Then they would prescribe a herb that ruled under the same astrological sign. Culpeper said that "He that would know the reason for the operation of the Herbs, must look up as high as the stars."

Medical practice started changing at the same time as Paracelsus and Culpeper were promoting signatures and astrology in conjunction with herbalism. Men such as Francis Bacon and William Harvey were changing science into an experimental process, leaving behind its speculative nature.

This was the point where biological and medical science started to separate from traditional herbalism. As the herbalists were trying to revive ancient practices, the medical scientists were starting to revolutionize the way science was perceived completely. This difference in purpose is what split medicine into two different categories.

From there, herbalists who refused to acknowledge the signatures and the stars but focused on classification started the science called Botany.

Physicians who taught Harvey's blood circulation theory was more useful than Cupeper's astrology theory, started what today we call scientific medicine.

The discoveries made in the middle ages by these exceptional men are considered milestones in the history of Western herbal medicine. From the main source, the ancient herbalists, to its drift from medical science.

Looking at how scientific medicine separated from traditional herbalism it's difficult to believe one of them might be wrong. Maybe it would have been better for experimental medicine to mix with the traditional herbalism and form a more comprehensive way of looking at healing. Something is certain, however, the fact that herbs play an important role in healing and their importance needs to be acknowledged in every part of the world.

Traditional herbalism has started to be seen as a method of alternative medicine in the United States and the Western world in general since 1910 when the Flexner Foundation released a document addressed to all medical institutions, defining the way medicine should be practiced and taught. The book was called the Flexner Report and it led all eclectic medical schools where botanical medicine was exclusively practiced, to close for good.

In the Eastern world, Mao Zedong reintroduced into the health care system the Traditional Chinese Medicine which relies heavily on herbalism, in 1949. Since then, the schools have been training thousands of practitioners in the basics of Chinese medicine, to practice it in hospitals. Hundreds of Americans fly to China to get an education in Chinese Medicine which shows us that there are many health practicers unhappy with the government's decision over a century ago.

In 1930 The UK was experiencing issues in the practice of herbalism, stemming from the difference from scientific medicine. The United States started prohibiting the practice around the same time. The World Health Organisations is estimating that about 80% of people rely on herbal medicine for some part of their health care. Germany has over 600 plant-based ones available and over 70% of physicians are prescribing them there.

Even though around the world the practice of prescribing treatments and medicines to patience is dependent on a medical license, no law prohibits the prescriptions or recommendation of plant-based remedies to anyone.

Looking at the world today, there is still a split between Western and Eastern medicine. In the Eastern world, and more specifically China, traditional herbalism is being preserved and used daily by the patients and prescribed by the doctors. It is a big part of their culture and their national pride.

The Western world is turning their back towards the practice and the scientists are focusing their efforts on experimental based medicine while forgetting often of the benefits plants have on the human body.

It might be worth looking at each culture and finding the benefits from each of their medical practices. One thing is certain though, herbal medicine still plays a very important role in most of the world's population and health.

Chapter 2
Popular Herbs Known to Improve Health

Herbs are embedded in the forefront of history. For hundreds of years, they have been fused into rich traditions and cultures all over the world. The medicinal properties of these plants are still very relevant today. You might have come across some of these popular herbs while walking through a garden or have some growing in your backyard. Here are some of those well-known herbs widely recognized for boosting health.

1. Burdock

- Scientific name: Arctium lappa
- Origin: although this plant is native to Asia and Europe, many species of burdock have been spread all over the world. Today, you can find it growing in fields, empty spaces, and roadsides across North America, China, Britain, Europe, and other continents.
- Description: the burdock fruit is rough and ovate with prickly heads. The burrs annoyingly cling to clothing and fur. The burdock plant is widely considered a weed in the United States but it is cultivated in Asia for the delicious root used in Korean and Chinese

delicacies. Some species of burdock can have their leaves grow up 28 inches long.

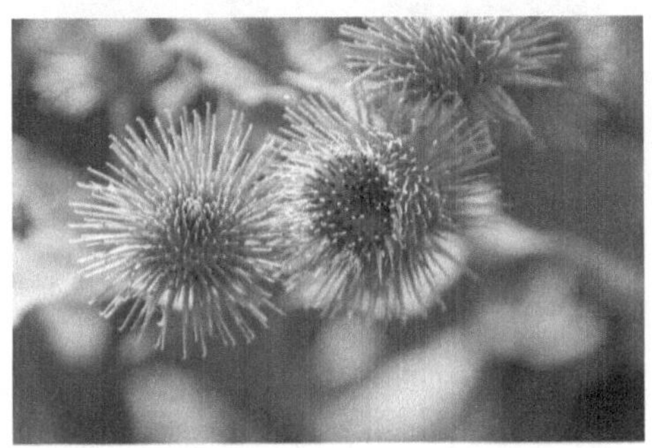

2. Calendula

- Scientific name: calendula officinalis
- Origin: the beautiful calendula flower is of northern Mediterranean origin. Its name is gotten from a Latin word 'kalendae' meaning the first day of a month. This is likely concerning the fact that calendulas bloom at the beginning of nearly every month of the year in local areas.
- Description: although calendula flowers are commonly called pot marigold, this herb should not be mistaken for plants in the marigold genus. Its bright golden yellow and orange color has been used for everything from fabric coloring to food and adorning statues in Hindu temples.

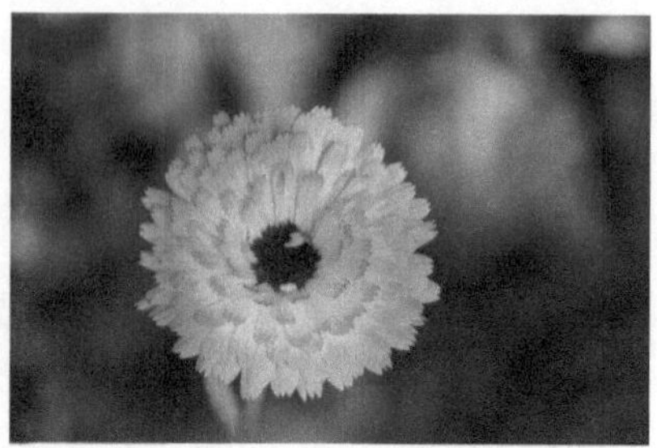

3. Chickweed

- Scientific name: Stellaria media
- Origin: chickweed originates from Eurasia in Europe but has now been naturalized all over the world.
- Description: is a perennial and annual flowering herb from the family Caryophyllaceae. It is a low growing plant with small leaves on erect stalks that can grow up to 18 inches tall. Chickweed yields white, small, star-shaped flowers almost all year round.

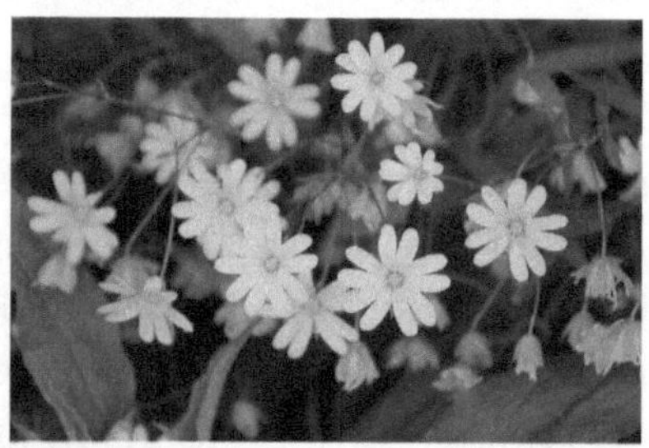

4. Dandelion

- Scientific name: Taraxacum officinale

- Origin: originally native to Eurasia, dandelions are now common in South America, North America, New Zealand, Australia, India, and many other regions that Europeans have migrated to. The English name is gotten from the French name 'dent de lion' meaning the lions tooth. This refers to the serrations like teeth on the plant's leaves.

- Description: Although many people assume dandelion is only a weed, it has been cultivated for herbal remedies for a long time. The leaves grow from the crown of the plant, they are basal. The stalk can grow up to 70cm tall and a milky latex oozes out if the stem is broken.

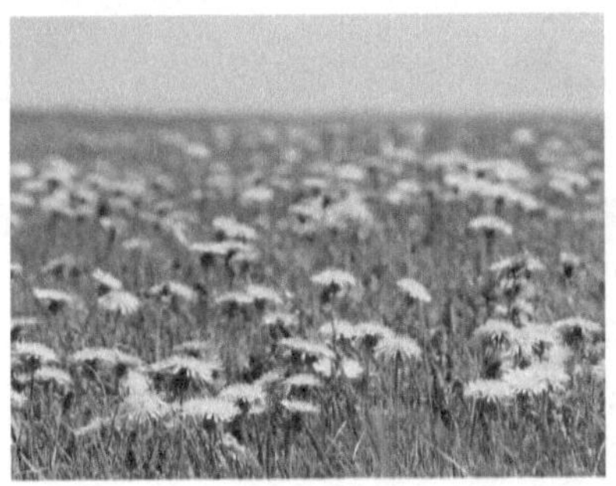

5. Echinacea

- Scientific name: Echinacea purpurea
- Origin: this flowering herb is indigenous to North America. Its earliest species can be traced back to Missouri and Arkansas from where it traveled towards the east in the 1970s. European

researchers made echinacea popular in 1939 when studies were carried out on aerial parts of the plant.

- Description: also known as coneflowers, echinacea is a flowering herb from the daisy family that has beautiful purple petals. The petals surround a cone or seed head made of dark brown or reddish spikes.

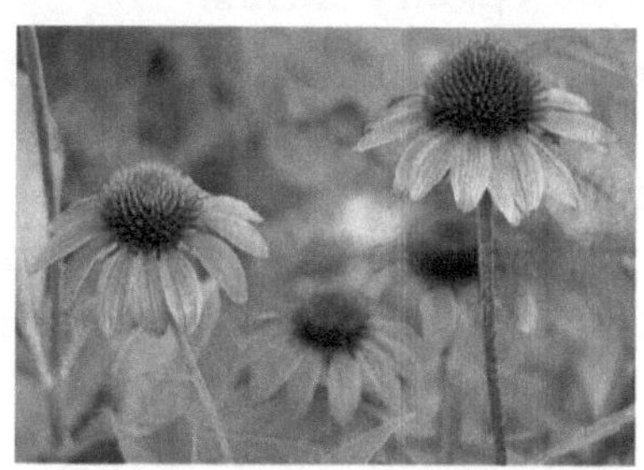

6. Elderflower

- Scientific name: Sambucus nigra cerulea
- Origin: this hedgerow plant is native to regions of Europe and Britain. The elder tree, from which elderflowers grow, is a fast-growing tree with flowers present from June to July and leaves from March to November each year. The history of elderflower goes back to the time of Greek physician Hippocrates in 400 BC.
- Description: the popularity of the elderflower plant has grown significantly in the past few years. Although there are rich history and many folklore about the herb, public interest in it peaked after it was announced as one of the ingredients for Prince Harry and Megan Markle's royal wedding cake.

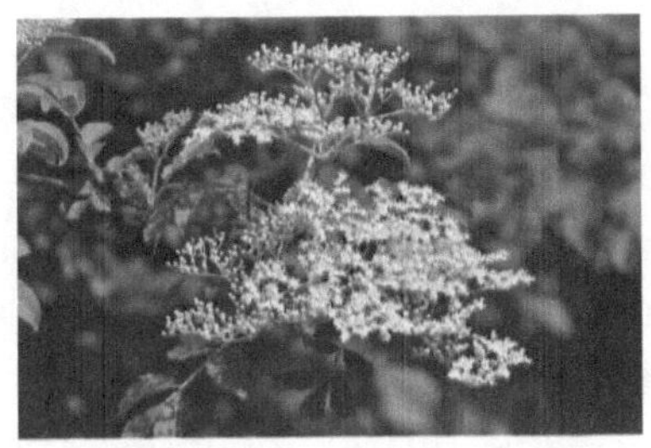

7. **Nettle**

- Scientific name: Urtica dioica
- Origin: this perennial flowering herb is native to Northern Africa, North America, Asia, and Europe. Nettle now grows all over the world especially in North America and New Zealand.
- Description: don't let the beautiful heart-shaped leaves fool you, nettle, or stinging nettle, can give you a bristly rash when your exposed skin brushes upon it. Its leaves and stems are covered with trichomes or stinging hairs that deliver chemical acids to cause the stinging sensation. Thankfully, this endearing plant loses its sting when boiled to release nutritious tonic effects.

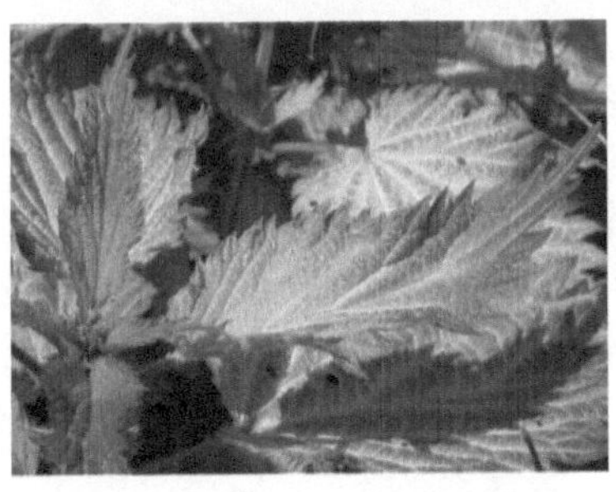

8. Oats

- Scientific name: Avena sativa
- Origin: probably originating from East Asia, oats date as far back as 2000 BC when they were weeds. They were first cultivated for medicinal purposes before they were grown for food. Today, they are widely farmed in many temperate areas.
- Description: bridging the divide between food and herbs, oats are a vintage restorative tonic. Oats, or wild oats, are from the grass family and one of the healthiest grains in the world. The annual plant can grow up to 5 feet tall. This tough plant can grow in sandy, highly acidic, low fertility soil provided there is sufficient water.

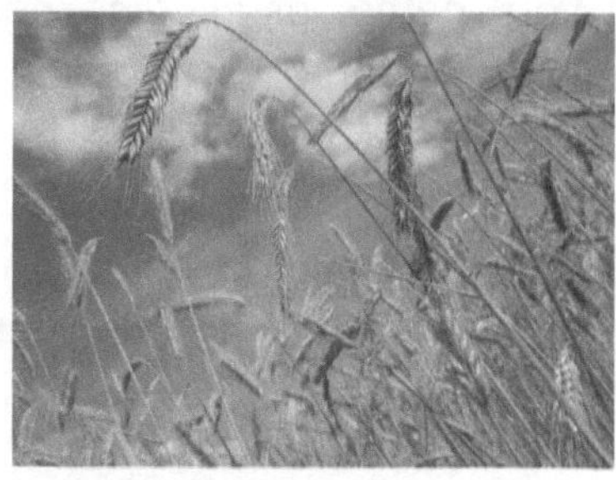

9. Peppermint

- Scientific name: Mentha x Piperita
- Origin: this hybrid herb is a cross between spearmint and watermint plants of the mint family originally from Asia and Europe. Peppermint is now widely

grown in many parts of the world and can also be found growing in the wild.

- Description: peppermint is highly valued for its flavor and it has many medicinal qualities as well. it features opposite growing leaves with jiggered edges and a crowning flower. Peppermint leaves can grow up to 3.5 inches tall while the purple flower only grows 0.31 inches tall. The flowering season for this aromatic herb lasts from mid-summer to late summer.

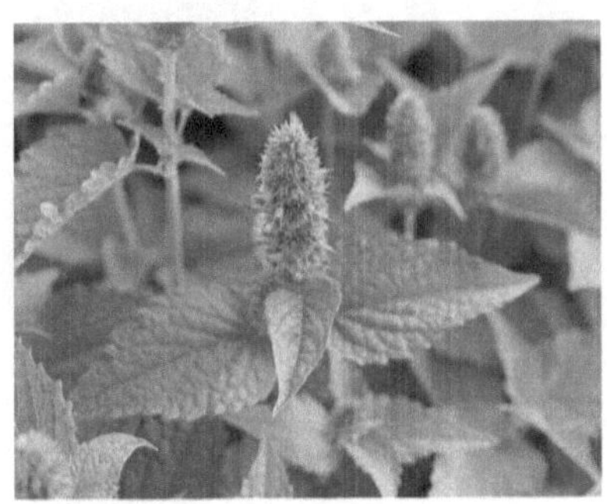

10. Yarrow

- Scientific name: Achillea millefolium
- Origin: this flowering plant of the aster family originated from the temperate regions of Western Asia and Europe but is now popularly grown in New Zealand, Australia, and North America. The name achillea is named after the Greek hero Achilles who

used the herb to treat the bleeding injuries of his Trojan War soldiers in 1200 BC.

- Description: this aromatic herb has foliage like fern and its name millefolium means a thousand leaves because yarrow leaves are finely partitioned. The plant has an erect, angular stem and lacy leaves that clasp under its simple stem. Its leaves can grow up to 6 inches tall.

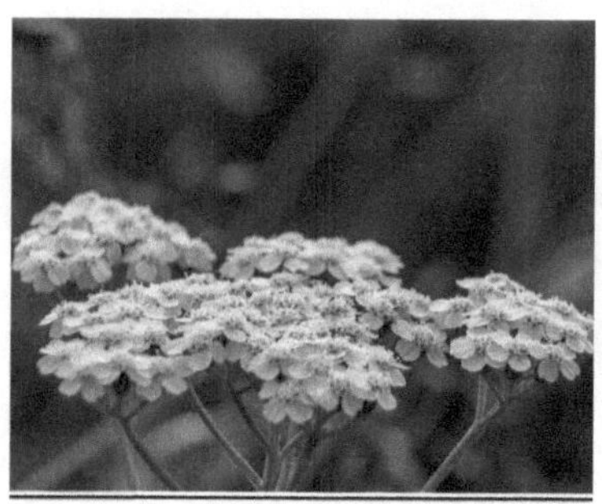

11. Cleavers

- Scientific name: Gallium aparine
- Origin: This amusing herb is a weed that can be found growing in fields across North America and Europe. Its nickname, bedstraw, came about because the plant was used as bedding. It is believed Mary added cleavers to Jesus' manger. Being a plant in the coffee family, cleaver seeds were roasted and substituted as coffee in local Sweden.

- Description: This climbing weed has long stalks and loopy leaves that easily fasten to other objects to facilitate the easy spreading of its seeds. It has been featured in traditional Chinese medication, native Indian remedies and is still used today as a diuretic.

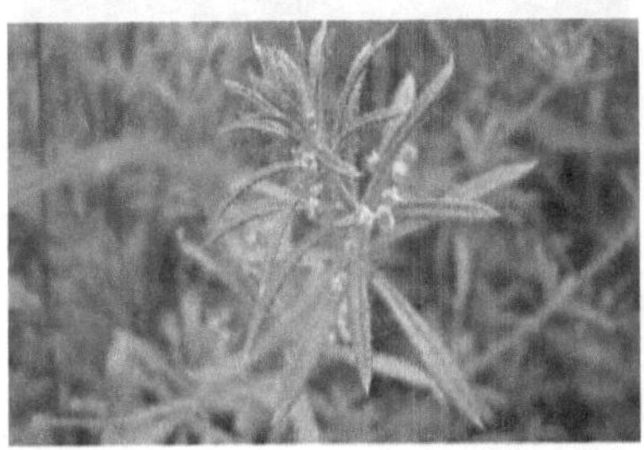

12. Gumweed

- Scientific name: Grindelia squarrosa
- Origin: this short-lived plant is native to central and western North America including California, New Mexico, Texas, British Columbia, and Quebec.
- Description: The gumweed herb blooms from July to the end of September producing many yellow ray flowers. It can be found growing in streamsides and roadsides. Gumweed has grey-green leaves and can grow up to 40 inches tall.

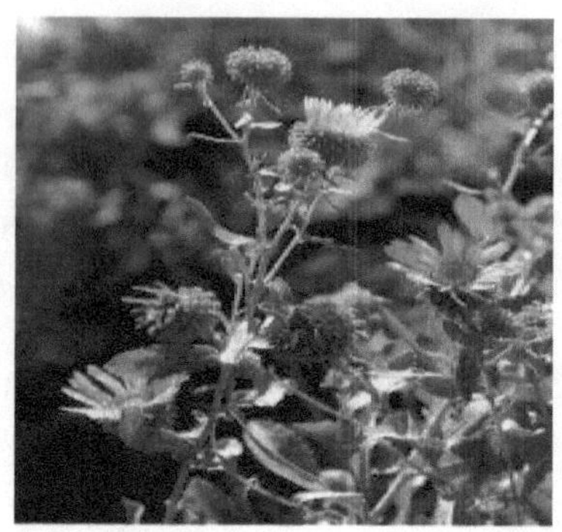

13. Fennel

- Scientific name: Foeniculum vulgare
- Origin: fennel now grows plentifully in many parts of the world but originally grew in the Mediterranean area. Its name is derived from the Latin word 'foeniculum' meaning little hay describing its feathery leaves. The name also refers to its conventional use in nurturing goats to boost the quality of their milk.
- Description: This perennial herb is from the carrot family. The flowery plant has feathery leaves and yellow flowers. Fennel mostly grows on dry soil near riverbanks and sea coasts. The pleasant-smelling herb looks and tastes like the plant anise but the two are very different.

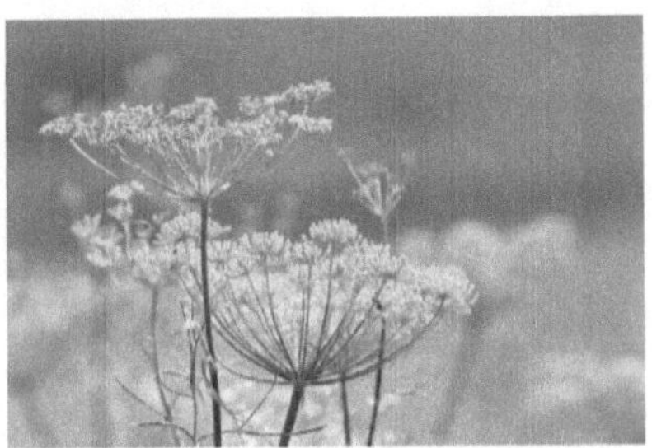

14. Mugwort

- Scientific name: Artemisia vulgaris
- Origin: this plant is indigenous to Asia and temperate Northern Europe but can be found in many regions of North America. Chinese songs from 3 BC mention this ancient herb.
- Description: this daisy family plant smells like sage, has bitter leaves, and an angular stem. It typically grows up to 4 feet but can easily climb to 6 feet. Its leaves are whitish under and dark green above. In the summer, mugwort blooms with a dark orange or yellow flowers. The mugwort plant is a tough survivor, it can be found growing in the most unlikely of places.

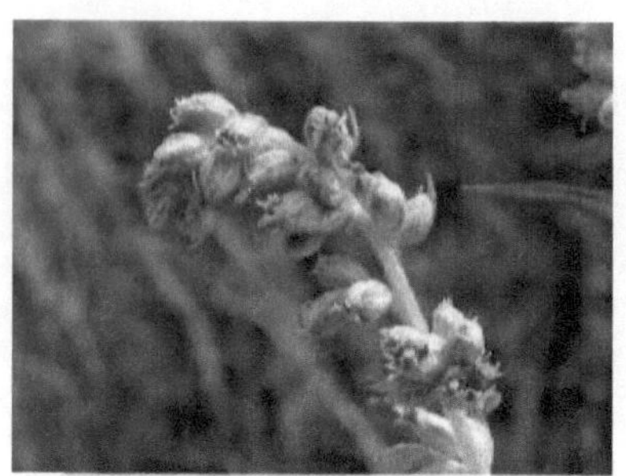

15. Mullein

- Scientific name: Verbascum thapsus
- Origin: the plant is indigenous to the Mediterranean, Asia, North Africa, and Europe. Today, it can be found in many parts of Australia and North America. Its name is derived from the Latin word 'mollis' meaning soft. Since the leaves have a very soft texture, we say this is a befitting name.
- Description: the golden yellow flowers of mullein are piled on a towering stalk across open spaces and fields all over the world. An oil infusion can be gotten from the sweet flowers. The leaves and flowers can be used as a dye and even the dried leaves aren't useless.

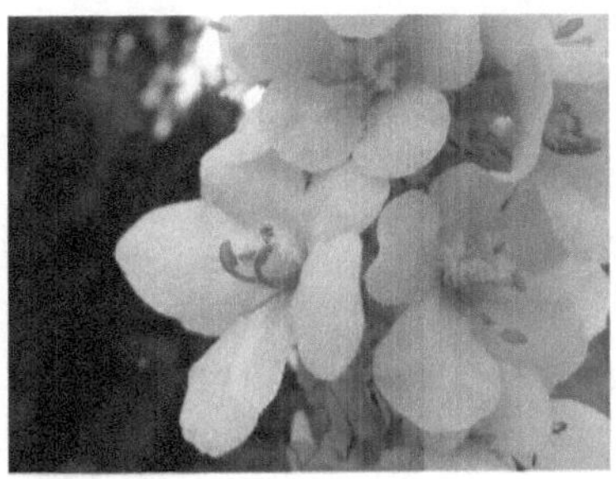

16. Yellow Dock

- Scientific name: Rumex Crispus
- Origin: this herb is native to Western Asia and Europe but now grows all over North America. Many native American tribes used yellow dock extensively for remedies from constipation to wound infection and yellow fever.
- Description: yellow dock has slender leaves that curl at the edges and fade away as they climb higher up the stem. The flowers are a green seed that turns brownish or deep red in the fall indicating it is time for harvest.

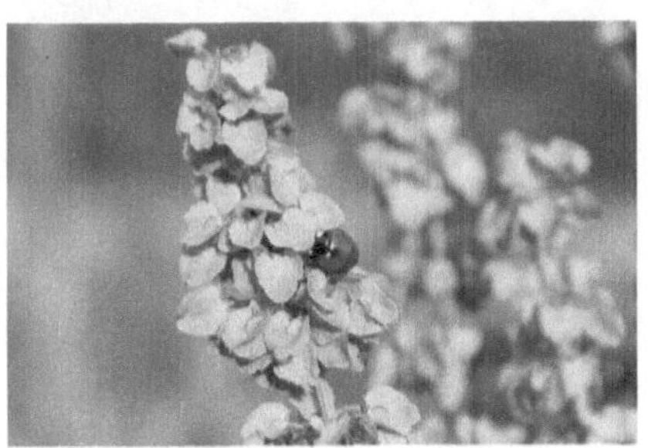

17. Parsley

- Scientific name: Petroselinum Crispus
- Origin: parsley is one of the most popular culinary herbs of all time. It originated from the Mediterranean areas of Tunisia, Algeria, and Southern Italy but is now widely grown throughout Europe and the United States. Greek mythology says parsley came from the blood of Archemorus, the forbearer of death. This flavor-enhancing, nutritious and medicinal food was probably associated with death because it has an uncanny resemblance to 'fool's parsley', a toxic plant also of Mediterranean origin.
- Description: because parsley is in the fennel and carrot family, it is no surprise the roots are edible. The taste of the root is bitter, not sweet but it is very nutritious. The curly leaves of the herb are also used as a food garnish as it enhances the fresh clean look of a dish.

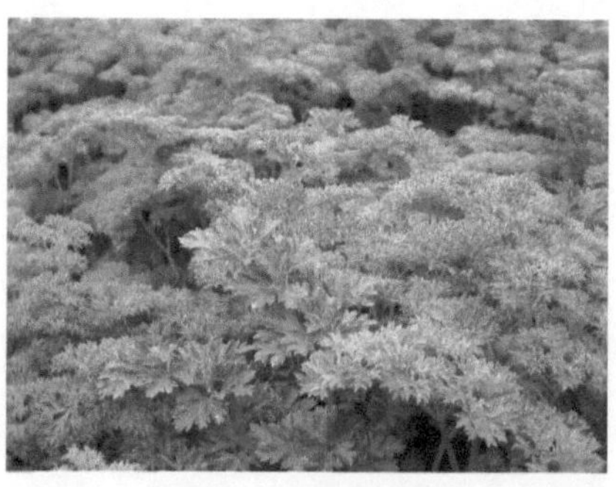

18. Chamomile

- Scientific name: Matricaria recutita
- Origin: chamomile originated in West Asia and Europe. From ancient times, the medicinal qualities of the herb have been valued by Romans, Egyptians, and Greeks. Many cultures considered the herb a god-sent plant. The name is gotten from the Latin word 'matrix' meaning womb. This refers to the soothing abilities it gives like that of a mother.
- Description: this group of daisy-like flowery plants from the Asteraceae family has been consumed for centuries and most popularly as a tea. It is used to treat a wide range of medical conditions but indigestion is the most popular.

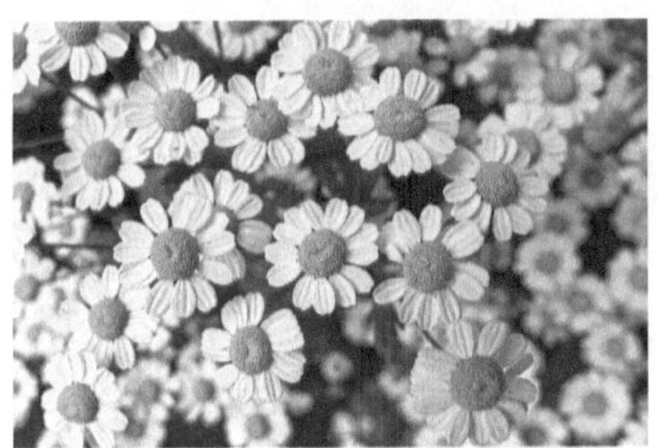

19. Holy Basil

- Scientific name: Ocimum sanctum
- Origin: the aromatic perennial herb is different from the Thai herb plant commonly used to flavor soups. Holy basil is indigenous to India but has been widely cultivated all over the tropics of Southeast Asia, West Africa, Australia, and some countries in the

Middle East. Ayurveda texts dating back to 1000 BC describe this leafy green plant as 'the incomparable one' and claim it is an embodiment of Tulasi, Lord Vishnu's consort.

- Description: holy basil is a small perennial shrub that can grow up to 3.3 feet tall. It has a peppery spicy flavor and is considered a sacred plant in Hinduism. The leaves are usually purple or green with a hairy stem and simple leaves growing in opposite directions along the stalk.

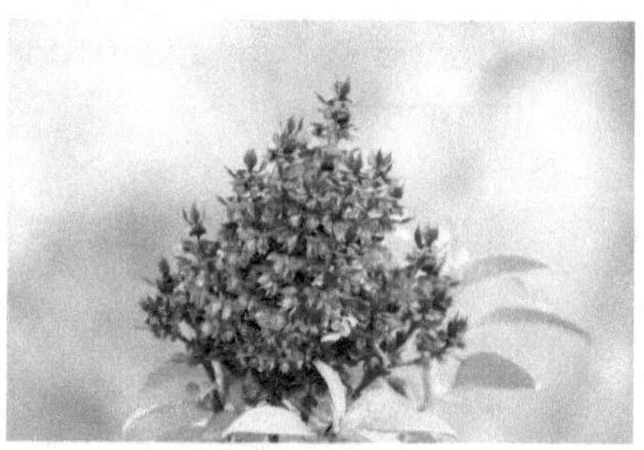

20. Fenugreek

- Scientific name: Trigonella foenum-graecum
- Origin: fenugreek is native to Western Asia, Southern Europe, and the larger Mediterranean region. Now, it is mostly cultivated in China, India, and the Middle East. In ancient times, fenugreek was used in Ayurvedic medicine, Chinese medicine, and European folk medicine.
- Description: the leaves, twigs, roots, and seeds of fenugreek are useful whether dried or fresh. It has a

cluster of three small obovate leaflets with a single stem less than 3 feet tall. The plant has a strong aroma and grows erect.

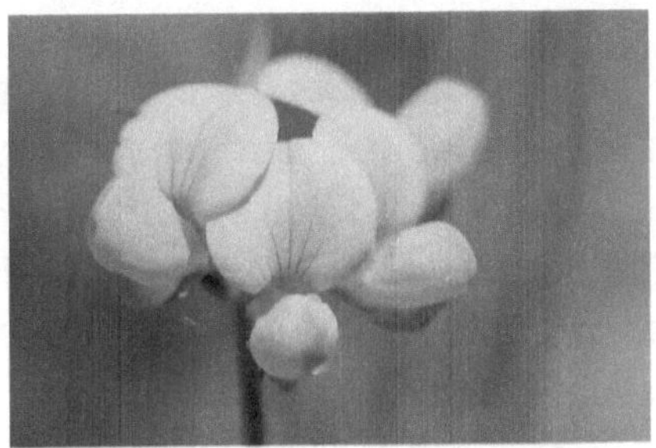

Whether you're a vegetarian, paleo dieter or you eat just about anything, you can find suitable herbs for your selection of food. Make a habit of eating herbs every day to improve your health and boost the nutrition of every meal. With so many of these herbs available, your taste buds will not be jaded. If you grow your herbs fresh or stock up from your local farmers market, you can enjoy the benefits of herbs all year round. Some of these plants can even be dried or frozen to extend their shelf life.

Chapter 3
Benefits of Common Herbs

Industrial pharmaceuticals and technological advancements have edged out powerful potions and elixirs for surgeries and pills when it comes to healthcare. Although this is the case, herbs have not lost their potency. People who want a stronger immune system, significant boosts in vitamins, and answers to varied ailments still opt for natural remedies found in herbs.

Many common herbs can be utilized for therapeutic and medicinal purposes. Take a look below at how the ordinary herbs you come in contact with every day can be helpful to you and your well-being.

1. Burdock

Burdock has been an active ingredient in conventional Chinese medicine for hundreds of years. Originally, it was mostly used to treat digestive and diuretic problems but modern-day research has found many possible uses for the herb.

- Skin conditions: when topically applied to the skin, the antibacterial properties in burdock helps fight skin conditions like acne, eczema, and psoriasis.

- Toxin removal: the herb is effective in riding the bloodstream of toxins. Burdock can detoxify the blood and promote better circulation.
- Antioxidants: burdock houses numerous potent antioxidants including luteolin, phenolic acids, and quercetin.

2. Calendula

There is mention of calendula being used in ancient Chinese and Ayurvedic medicine. The sunny blooms of calendula are effective as a wound healing, anti-inflammatory, antimicrobial herb to remedy all manner of skin issues.

- Skin healing: oil can be extracted from the calendula flower for topical use in treating wounds, sunburns, bruises, rashes, stings, and insect bites. You can also make a salve from the herb and use it to treat eczema, acne, swellings, and cold sores. It can also be used on cervical dysplasia and yeast infections.
- Other benefits: the herb is edible and can be used in food, salads, and tea as a soothing ingredient. A yellow dye can be extracted from the flowers and used on food or fabric.

3. Chickweed

In ancient times, the leaves, flowers, and stem of chickweed were used teas, extracts, and decorations. The powerful plant components in this herb are the reason for its benefits.

- Skin conditions: when rubbed topically, chickweed can treat itchy skin, rashes, wounds, burns, contact dermatitis, eczema, and psoriasis. It can even be used against nappy rash in babies.
- Weight loss: when properly administered, chickweed could help fight obesity-induced by progesterone.

4. Dandelion

This herb is a pesky weed for most people but native Americans and ancient Chinese healers used dandelion to treat liver and stomach conditions. Dandelion root, fresh or dried, can be used to make tinctures, teas, and poultices.

- Skin damage: dandelion can be dried, ground, and made into a paste by adding some water. This soothes skin problems like eczema, acne, rashes, psoriasis, and boils. Its antipruritic and anti-inflammatory qualities can also help stop sun damage.
- Liver damage: when consumed as a tonic, dandelion cleanses the liver, relieving it of stress and makes room for liver regeneration.

- Blood pressure: research shows that the diuretic effects of dandelion can be useful in treating premenstrual bloating, prediabetes, and water retention.

5. Echinacea

The purple coneflower isn't popular for no reason. This herb is packed full of benefits know to fight problems of inflammation, pain, flu, migraines, and others.

- Skin concerns: the anti-bacterial and anti-inflammatory properties of echinacea impede the growth of Propionibacterium, acne-causing bacteria. When applied topically, echinacea also helps reduce wrinkles, hydrate skin, and enhance the symptoms of eczema.
- Cancer: this herb is useful in suppressing the growth of cancer cells and possibly triggers the death of cancer cells too.
- Reduces anxiety: echinacea contains caffeic acid, rosmarinic, and alkamides that are all helpful in fighting anxiety.

6. Elderflower

Although elderflower is more widely used for its flavoring, the herb has many medicinal benefits. Elderflower has antioxidant, anti-inflammatory, anti-cancer, and antimicrobial properties useful for fighting diseases.

- Respiratory illnesses: the anti-inflammatory and antiseptic properties of elderflower make it ideal for fighting the flu, sinus infections, colds, and other respiratory illnesses.
- Laxative and diuretic: elderflower can help ease constipation.
- Boost immune system: its antiviral and antibacterial properties are useful for fighting allergies and boosting the immune system.
- Wounds: it can be used to stop bleeding from injuries.
- Blood sugar: elderflower can work like insulin to reduce blood sugar levels.

7. Nettle

Stinging nettle has been helpful for herbal remedies since ancient times. Roman soldiers massaged it into their skin to keep warm and Egyptians used it to treat back pain and arthritis. Nettle has many nutrients including vitamin A, several B vitamins, vitamins C, and K, all the essential amino acids, sodium, iron, calcium, and more.

- Reduce inflammation: the herb has properties that can help your body fight inflammation.
- Hay fever: nettle shows a lot of promise for treating hay fever. It stops inflammations that trigger allergies.
- Controls blood sugar: nettle is linked to lowering blood sugar in humans and animals alike.

8. Oats

Oats are a gluten-free superfood rich with minerals, vitamins, antioxidants, and fiber. The plant has been cultivated for medicinal remedies long before it was grown as a food.

- Contains beta-glucan: this fiber is useful for reducing blood sugar levels, reducing cholesterol, increasing good bacteria, and making you feel fuller for longer.
- Protects from cholesterol damage: because of the high quantity of beta-glucan in oats, cholesterol circulation is reduced in your body when you eat oats.
- Weight loss: because oats are very filling, it can help with weight loss in the long run.
- Skincare: finely ground oats help protect the skin, treat itching, and reduce irritation.

9. Peppermint

Romans, Greeks, and Egyptians used peppermint for medicine centuries ago. You can use the herb as an extract, a tea, or an oil.

- Relieves stomach upset: doctors recommend peppermint for alleviating nausea and vomiting as well as other stomach discomforts.
- Irritable bowel symptoms: peppermint capsules are used to treat constipation, gas, and diarrhea.
- Headache: the menthol in peppermint can lessen migraines and headaches.
- Mouth germs: peppermint is known as a breath freshener and its antibacterial properties help to kill the source of bad breath too.
- Energy boost: peppermint oil can chase sleep and dullness away to give you a boost during work.

10. Yarrow

From the time of the Trojan War, this daisy herb has not been forgotten.

- Toothache: chewing the fresh leaves of yarrow herb has been known to reduce toothache.
- Healing effect: yarrow oil is infused in shampoos and other products to induce a soothing, healing effect.

- Wound bleeding: yarrow promotes sweating to halt bleeding from wounds. It is even used to alleviate heavy bleeding from menstrual cycles.

11. Cleavers

From ancient times, cleavers has acted as a diuretic in herbal medicine. It has been used to treat bladder infections by promoting urine and relieving edema. The aerial parts of cleaver herb are used by modern-day herbalists to:

- Support the lymphatic glands. Taking cleavers promotes natural detoxification of the body.
- Support mucosal membrane health of the skin and urinary tracts.

12. Gumweed

This herb is a fantastic natural muscle relaxant. Favored for its medicinal qualities by many tribes of Native Americans, gumweed is commonly used to treat bronchial problems and asthma.

- Lung problems: this herb helps to relax and open your airways to relieve problems like asthma and bronchitis. It also helps eliminate phlegm and catarrh so that breathing is improved.
- Calming: gumweed reduces the reactivity of nerve endings inside your bronchial tube so that the heart rate is reduced and the person is calmed.
- Skin problems: when used as a topical treatment, gumweed can address problems like burns, boils, poison ivy rash, insect bites, and dermatitis.

13. Fennel

The bulb of the fennel plant has a licorice flavor but this flavor is stronger in the seed since it contains some oil. Aside from the culinary uses of fennel, the herb has many health benefits you can enjoy.

- Reduce menstrual pain: women who take fennel extracts daily experience less menstrual cramps than women who don't.

- Weight control: fennel makes you feel fuller without adding extra calories. It also helps secret anethole to help with appetite control.
- Relieves constipation: many cultures use fennel as a laxative to ease the passing of stool during constipation.

14. Mugwort

Because the mugwort plant grows aggressively and can take over whole spaces in a short while, people treat and destroy it as a weed. However, mugwort is known to reduce itching, promote blood circulation, boost energy, and support a healthy liver.

- Diuretic: it deals with fluid retention by increasing a person's urine output.
- Better menstrual cycles: it acts as an emmenagogue and promotes regular, uniform menstrual cycles.
- Calms nerves: is widely used as a nervine.
- Others: mugwort is used in treating numerous health problems including colic, fatigue, epilepsy, headache, constipation, vomiting, hypochondria, and restlessness.

15. Mullein

Some compounds found in the flowers and leaves of this herb act as expectorants or demulcents. Because of this, mullein can calm skin inflammations and irritations of some internal parts.

- Ear infections: when used as an active ingredient in eardrops, mullein is effective in dealing with ear pain and otalgia.
- Flu: mullein attacks viruses that cause the flu and prevent serious illnesses that arise from the flu including pneumonia.
- Others: herbalists also utilize mullein in treating coughs, asthma, bronchitis, and infections in the upper respiratory tract.

16. Yellow dock

Yellow dock is a wonderful herb for modern-day natural remedies. Among many uses, it is beneficial in liver detoxification and healthy digestion.

- Blood detoxification: it is used for cleansing and detoxifying the blood.
- Diarrhea: drinking yellow dock is a popular cure for malaria and diarrhea.
- Fever: the herb is loaded with manganese, vitamin A and phosphorus, all effective medication for fever.

- Anemia: because yellow dock cleanses the blood, it has been used to heal anemia.
- Throat disorders: the yellow dock is popularly known for its sore throat and gut treating properties.

17. Parsley

Parsley is not your regular garnish. The herb contains iron, calcium, vitamin C, vitamin K, and many antioxidant compounds useful fighting several ailments.

- Allergies: you can extract essential oils from parsley leaves to help treat seasonal allergies by suppressing inflammation.
- Diabetes: it was found that parsley is effective in tackling liver damage caused by diabetes. The herb is full of antioxidants that make it strong enough to fight diabetes.
- Breast cancer: parsley produces apigenin, a non-toxic chemical for treating cancer. Apigenin is known for reducing the tumor size of aggressive breast cancer.

18. Chamomile

Chamomile is very popular as an aid for sleep but it is useful for dealing with anxiety too.

- Anxiety: clinical trials with chamomile indicate it has subtle anti-anxiety effects on people suffering from anxiety disorders.
- Insomnia: added to its anti-anxiety properties, chamomile is also a light sedative that can induce sleep when administered in the right amount.
- Digestive problems: chamomile stops the growth of stomach ulcer-causing bacteria. It is also useful for reducing stomach muscle spasms.
- Oral health: the anti-inflammatory and antimicrobial properties of chamomile make it effective against plaque and gingivitis when used as a mouthwash.

19. Holy Basil

This medicinal herb packs a lot of health-boosting effects including anti-inflammatory, antimicrobial, antioxidant, antidiarrheal, anticoagulant, anti-diabetic, anti-arthritic, and more.

- Chronic illness: the Ayurvedic practice of ingesting a certain amount of holy basil every day has been proven to help fight a host of present-day chronic sicknesses.
- Inflammation: many studies have pointed to holy basil as an effective tool against numerous illnesses associated with inflammation. The herb can work

alone or with other substances to impede inflammation.

- Other applications: holy basil has many other medicinal benefits including the treatment of stress, anxiety, fever, back pain, ringworm, malaria, dysentery, asthma, snakebites, and heart disease.

20. Fenugreek

Although fenugreek seeds are bitter, this plant can be used against a host of medical problems.

- Diabetes: the chemicals and fiber contained in fenugreek slow the absorption of carbohydrates and sugar. This increases the body's insulin level.
- Boost fertility: men who regularly take fenugreek experienced a boost in testosterone, libido, and strength.
- Prevent cancer: the plant contains phytochemicals useful in fighting cancers.
- Aid nursing mothers: Ayurvedic medicine recommends fenugreek to increase milk quality in breastfeeding mothers.

Take note that this is not an exhaustive list, not even close. Each medicinal property of every herb discussed above is very real and can oftentimes be boosted by combining herbs. Blends of herbs can form ointments, teas, and tinctures with increased healing potential for your body. Always make sure to use organic products that are homegrown or bought from reputable sources. This ensures the quality of your end products and guarantees effectiveness. Also, be sure to consult with your healthcare professional before concocting herb mixtures for personal treatment.

Chapter 4
Tea Recipes

As a species, humans regularly make sure to cook with herbs, however, utilizing them in refreshments can be similarly as accomplishing. Other than having astonishing aromas, the therapeutic properties of herbs are in some cases intensified with the expansion of boiling water.

An assortment of herbal tea mixes is accessible for purchasing, yet regularly these business mixes utilize fake flavorings and are not the genuine piece by any stretch of the imagination. You can maintain a good distance from these by making your own mixes utilizing characteristic flowers and herbs you have grown or gathered yourself. Blending your herbs for tea is as simple as picking the fragrances that intrigue you and mixing up your preferred decisions. In summer, you may favor a scrumptious frosted tea, while winter may see you fermenting a decent warm tea to avoid the chill.

First of all, herbal tea may help battle colds by clearing nasal entries and halting substantial hacks. This is additionally said to lessen asthma. Herbal tea is known to help assimilation/digestion. It can help split down fats and accelerate the purging of the stomach, which will lessen the side effects of swelling, acid reflux, and heaving. The best teas for this are dandelion, peppermint, ginger, and chamomile. Herbal tea contains cancer prevention agents that may bring down the danger of ceaseless illness. The best teas for this are echinacea, ginger, elderberry, and yarrow root. Here are some of the tea recipes which you can easily prepare at home.

Hot Burdock Tea

Due to its medicinal properties, Burdock Herb, scientifically known as, *Artium lappa,* can be easily made into tea. It can either be sliced or directly be added to soups and broths. Initially, it was used purely as a medicinal herb and had been effective in curing, measles, cold, sore throat, arthritis, and many other common diseases like tonsillitis, etc. But now the National Institute of Health in the USA has recently claimed that Burdock might have beneficial effects on human health. Recent studies show that Burdock might have a cure for HIV, bacterial infections, cancer, and kidney stones. But make sure to consult health care professionals before using any kind of herb as a permanent medicine.

Ingredients:

- 2 cups of water
- Fresh or dried burdock root
- Stainless-steel teapot

Procedure:

i.   First, select a fresh burdock root. Keep in mind that these will not stay fresh for long and often will start to rot. So, if there are some leftover Burdock roots, you can add them to some curry or soup.

ii. In case you have selected a purely fresh root you can simply wipe the dirt with a clean cloth. On the other hand, if you have picked a bit older root you can clean the burdock root by scrapping off the edges with a knife.

iii. In case you don't have a fresh root, you can also use a tablespoon of dried burdock root powder.

iv. Add evenly chopped pieces of the root to the teapot and add 3 to 4 cups of filtered water. Heat thoroughly till the water boils and then lower the heat to let it constantly cook on low heat for at least 2 to 30 minutes. This will extract out all the essence of the herb.

v.   Serve the tea hot. You can store and consume the tea as a detox throughout the day. But remember that burdock is a diuretic so do not over-consume.

<u>Fresh Calendula Tea</u>

Calendula is also an ancient herb and is regularly used in tea. Due to its vast uses, the herb is very famous and is quite well-known for its therapeutic use. The tea can be utilized as a gargle for sore throat. It can also be used as an anti-inflammatory agent and can be applied to ruptured skin. You can easily wash your face for its anti-acne properties. Pouring some on the foot could also cure athletes' foot. Or it could also be used as a rinsing agent if you have itchy eyes. While all these are the external uses of the tea, it is also reported to have cured gastric ulcers and sore throat. It can also help break a high fever by sweating. But you must consult your physician before using it as any kind of proper medication if you have chronic conditions because it can also intensify bleeding in menstruation and pregnant women should consult their gynecologists first.

Ingredients

- 2 – 3 Cups of freshwater.
- Fresh Calendula Flowers
- Stainless-steel teapot

Procedure

i. If you have picked it fresh, then you can simply add the flowers to the teapot after washing them with tap water and carry on with the next step. In the case of dried flowers, mash dried flowers and grind them.
ii. Add 1 to 2 tablespoons of the mashed calendula powder to the teapot.
iii. Add 3 to 4 cups of freshwater to the teapot.
iv. Cover the pot and let the water boil.
v. After boiling, leave the pot on low heat to extract all the aroma of the herb. This will make the tea more concentrated. If you want to keep it light. Just pull it off a bit earlier.

vi.   Serve it hot. Or you can simply let infuse until it cools down. You can store it and consume it throughout the day.

Chickweed Herbal Tea

Chickweed tea has been utilized as a home-grown cure since the sixteenth century assisting with respiratory issues as well as skin maladies and aggravations. This tea (to be taken in) would be prescribed to those with poor assimilation and even to those experiencing tuberculosis. The chickweed herb contains various vitamins and minerals. It is rich in Vitamin B, B-complex, A, and C. It also contains calcium, zinc, potassium, flavonoids, and iron along with many other nutrients. All these essential vitamins and minerals make this a healthy beverage to be included in your weekly diet plan. It can cure skin and tissue problems, can act as a blood purifier, help you in losing weight, and be used as a natural sedative.

Ingredients:

- 2 to 3 cups of water
- The aerial part of chickweed plant
- Stainless-steel teapot

Procedure:

i.   This recipe will start by boiling water in the teapot. Start heating 2 to 3 cups of water until it boils.

ii.   Now we will add the chickweed herb to the cups. If you have dried chickweed, add 1 tablespoon to the cups. In case you have fresh herb then add 2 tablespoons to each cup.

iii.   If you have taken fresh herb, then remember to cut the leaves to let the flavor out.

iv.   Once the water has boiled, add it hot into the cups and let the herb steep for 5 to 10 minutes.

v.   You can also add honey to the tea to even enhance the flavor.

vi.   Serve it hot.

Dandelion Tea

Many people know dandelion as a backyard weed, but if you look at its health benefits it proves to be a very beneficial flower. Dandelion tea can have many positive effects on your digestive system. It improves appetite and soothes digestive diseases. It also cures the detoxification of the liver. Dandelion tea acts as a natural diuretic and can flush out excess fluid from the body. Moreover, the tea is packed with loads of antioxidants that prevent the body from all types of cell damage and keeps the body and skin fresh.

Ingredients

- 2 – 3 cups of water
- Fresh dandelion flowers
- 2-3 Tablespoon of dried stevia leaf
- 3-4 limes (juiced)

Procedure

i.   The first step is to pick fresh dandelions. Pick only yellow parts of the flower and pull off any excess leaves which can be later used in salads etc.

ii.   Wash/Rinse with cold water thoroughly.

iii.   Take the water in the stainless-steel pot and start to heat. Heat till the water boils.

iv.   Add dandelion flowers to the boiling water. Cover the lid and let the flavor steep for 15 to 20 minutes.

v.   Add lime juice and stir well.

vi.   Serve it cold or at room temperature.

vii.   You can also store it to use throughout the day.

<u>Mint - Echinacea Tea</u>

Echinacea tea is a home-grown beverage most generally produced using the *Echinacea purpura* plant. Echinacea is a well-known solution for influenza, colds, and many different diseases. A few people additionally accept that echinacea can reduce torment, forestall malignancy, improve psychological wellness, and diminish a lot of skin issues. In any case, mainstream researchers and doctors do not concede to the advantages of echinacea tea and some have communicated concerns for echinacea symptoms. The flavor of echinacea tea is frequently portrayed as tongue-shivering. Truth be told, some home-grown item producers view this quality as proof of the herb's adequacy. Echinacea is usually joined with mint or with different fixings, for example, lemongrass to make an increasingly lovely tasting tea.

Ingredients

- 2 – 3 cups of water
- Dried echinacea leaves
- 1 tsp lemongrass (dried)
- 1 tsp mint (dried)

Instructions

i. Grind the ingredients and mix the three.
ii. Add water to the heating teapot and let it boil.
iii. Add all the mixed herbs in the boiling water.
iv. Allow the mixture to settle as it will steep for about 15 minutes. This will help the flavor ooze out and mix in water.
v. Enjoy plain or with honey. You can also enhance the flavor by adding other sweeteners.

Elderflower Tea

It is a disgrace that elderflower tea isn't well known yet since this herbal tea is exceptionally valuable. Additionally, it is heavenly in flavor, and smooth. Elderflower tea has a lot of benefits. It is also said to contain high levels of multiple vitamins. Most common of which is Vit C, due to which it can act as a powerful antioxidant. The herb is supposed to strengthen the heart and the immune system. Elderflower does support the metabolism and calms the stomach. It can also soothe stomach cramps. Additionally, it purifies the blood and also stimulates kidney activity.

Ingredients:

- 2 – 3 Cups of Fresh Water
- Elderflower (Dried or Fresh)
- Stainless – steel teapot.

Procedure:

i. To make elderflower tea from fresh or dried elderflowers just pick a few flower bunches of the fresh plant. If you have dried leaves, you can grind them to use in the next step.

ii. If taking fresh flowers you need to carefully cut all the stems as they are not safe to consume. They can be toxic.

iii. Fill the teapot with water and set it to heat, till it boils.

iv. Place the flower petals or 1 teaspoon of dried powder in the cup and pour the hot water.

v. Cover the lid and let the mixture settle for 15 to 20 minutes.

vi. Enjoy your fresh pot of elderflower tea. You can also add honey for further sweetening.

Nettle Herb Tea

Nettle is a shrub that is mainly found in Europe and Asia. Scientifically called *Urtica dioica*, nettle shrub has a lot of medicinal properties and can be used as herbal medicine. You can make it into a tea, which not only tastes good but can also cure urinal tract infections as well as being a delicious additive to your soups. Moreover, Nettle shrub has been used widely for curing arthritis pain and sore muscles, Some studies were done back in 2013, show that nettle leaf extract lowers the blood sugar levels in type 2 diabetic persons. Recipe for making delicious Nettle tea is as follows:

Ingredients:

- 2 - 3 cups of drinking water
- Nettle leaves (fresh or dries powder)
- Stainless-steel teapot

Procedure:

i. Add water to the teapot and set it to heat.
ii. Add 2 to 3 nettle leaves or 1 tablespoon nettle leaf powder if you have dry powder.
iii. Let the mixture heat for 15 to 20 minutes on low flame.
iv. When the water is about to boil, turn off the stove and let it sit for 5 to 10 minutes.
v. Add honey to the cups for sweetening the tea. You can also add cinnamon or stevia for assed flavors.

<u>Oats Tea</u>

Oats are wealthy in solvent filaments which help in bringing down cholesterol levels. These dissolvable strands help increment intestinal travel time and decrease glucose ingestion. Oats additionally contain beta-glucan which is a lipid bringing down the operator. Oats can also serve to be an extremely solid breakfast alternative. Be it a handy solution for cravings for food, light, and healthy night nibble or strong energy providing substance that helps you through your rushed morning, oats are simply the one superfood that can undoubtedly meet itself to suit your requirements. Oat teas have all the important nutrients one can include in a balanced diet.

Ingredients:

- 2 – 3 cups of water.
- 2 TB rolled oats
- 1 cinnamon stick
- Honey (more or less to taste)
- 2 tsp pure vanilla extract (more or less to taste)

Procedure:

i. Take a saucepan and put 2 to 3 cups of water in it.
ii. Put oats, cinnamon stick, into the saucepan and bring up to a boil.
iii. Turn the heat down and cover the lid for about 30 minutes.
iv. Turn off heat and add honey and vanilla.
v. Strain to remove oats if desired.

vi.   Serve hot.

<u>Peppermint Tea</u>

Peppermint frames a significant piece of our lives; from giving our irritated stomach some help to giving our beverages an invigorating taste and fragrance. Its calmative properties can leave you simply relaxed, and in mental peace. You may have known about peppermint tea that makes for a brilliant taste and having immense health and beauty benefits. Some peppermint teas can help you reduce weight. It also helps in relieving stomach acidity, lessens acid reflux, makes your skin gleam, initiates rest, and gives satiety, further helping you to get in shape. There is scarcely any symptom of peppermint tea; so, you can drink it whenever you need to.

Ingredients:

- 2 to 3 tablespoon crushed (fresh) peppermint leaves or dried leaves
- 3 – 4 cups of drinking water.
- Stainless-steel Pots

Procedure:

i.   The first step is to pick fresh leaves. Crush the leaves to make it easily mixable.

ii.   Wash/Rinse with cold water thoroughly.

iii.   Take the water in the stainless-steel pot and start to heat. Heat till the water boils.

iv.   Add the crushed peppermint leaves to the boiling water. Cover the lid and let the flavor steep for 15 to 20 minutes.

v.   Add lime juice and stir well.

vi.   Serve it hot, cold, or at room temperature.

vii.   You can also store it to use throughout the day.

Yarrow Tea

Yarrow is a long-stemmed member of the sunflower family. Yarrow tea can have many positive effects on your digestive system. It improves appetite and soothes digestive diseases. It also cures menstrual problems. Yarrow tea acts as a natural diuretic and can flush out excess fluid from the body and also fights bacteria, helping your immune system to stay strong. Moreover, the tea is packed with loads of antioxidants that prevent the body from all types of cell damage and keeps the body and skin fresh.

Ingredients

- 2 – 3 cups of water
- Fresh Yarrow flowers
- 3-4 limes (juiced)

Procedure

i. The first step is to pick fresh Yarrow. Pick only white parts of the flower and pull off any excess leaves.
ii. Wash/Rinse with cold water thoroughly.
iii. Take the water in the stainless-steel pot and start to heat. Heat till the water boils.
iv. Add Yarrow flowers to the boiling water. Cover the lid and let the flavor steep for 15 to 20 minutes.
v. Add lime juice and stir well.
vi. Serve it cold or at room temperature.
vii. You can also store it to use throughout the day.

Chapter 5
Making Your Own Tinctures

What Is A Tincture?

The universe of plants is an incredible one. There is an abundance of segments in plants that serve to ensure them at different phases of innovation, as there are such a significant number of forces at play including climate, predators (counting us), and soil quality. At the point when we expend these plant constituents in different structures, we can likewise receive the rewards – however, figuring out how to set up these plants and herbs appropriately isimportant.. This is the place handcrafted tinctures and tonics come in.

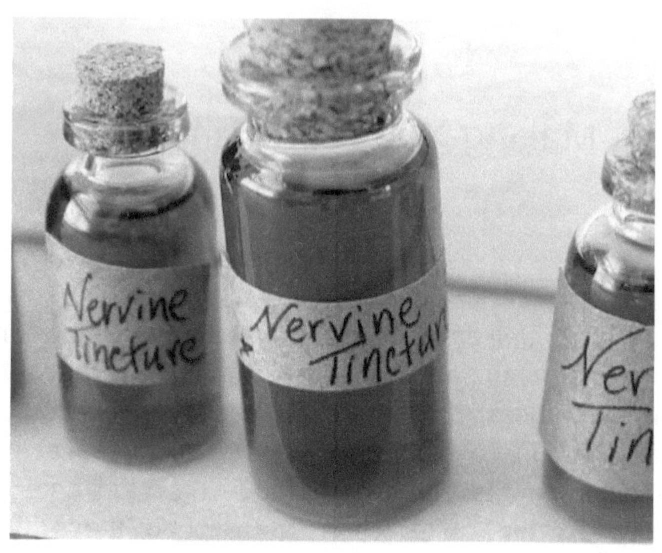

For quite a long time, herbalists have been creating mixtures of tinctures to fix regular sicknesses. Regardless of whether you need assistance in the digestive system, relaxation, or a stimulating lift to begin your day, there is probably a herb that can help. Herbs can be utilized dried or fresh to make tinctures. Fresh herbs have a more grounded fragrance, yet are not as powerful as dried herbs. Fresh herbs can add an aroma to the tincture, but dried herbs are clinically more beneficial.

Tinctures make it simple to consume the normal immunity-boosting substances found in certain plants. They are typically reasonably quick to make and can be effectively arranged at home. The availability of herbal cures like tinctures is most likely a significant motivation behind why an expected 80 percent of the total population depends on these medicines for a portion of their health needs. Tinctures are easy to make and are as beneficial as any other herbal tea. At the point when you need a prompt reaction, for example, herbs for immediate relaxation, a tincture may give you increasingly quick outcomes. For nutritive herbs that can take a little while of consumption to get results, either a tincture or a tea would be fine. It all depends on one's individual preference. Some commonly known Tinctures which can be readily made at home are described.

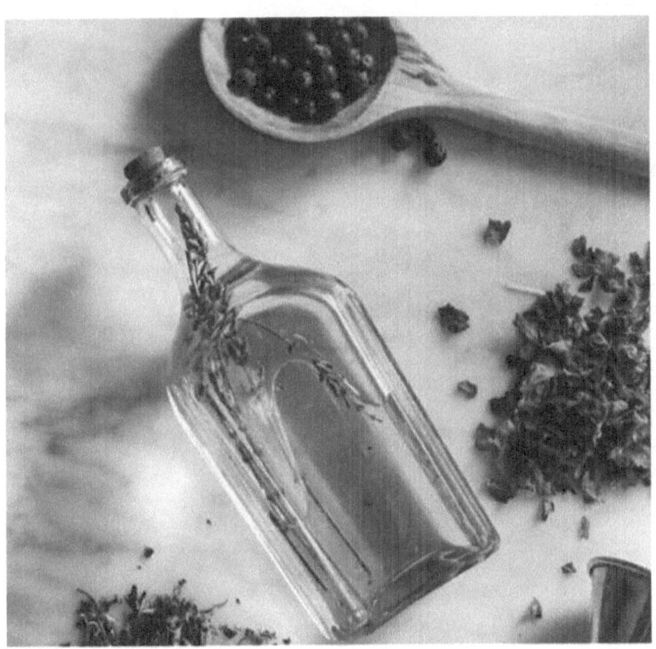

A tincture is only a concentrated herbal mixture made with liquor, which can be taken straight or diluted in tea or water. So, it is another method of removing the dynamic parts from a herb, with the exception that you are utilizing alcohol instead of vinegar, water, or any other dissolvable. Due to the alcohol in tinctures, the extracts of the herbs readily absorb into the blood and the effects are visible within an hour. Due to their active assimilation, tinctures prove to be the best treatment for things like stomach problems, pain, anxiety, and other sleep-related disorders. Commonly people utilize tinctures for the following diseases.

- Stress/anxiety
- Cold/flu
- Indigestion
- Allergies
- Insomnia

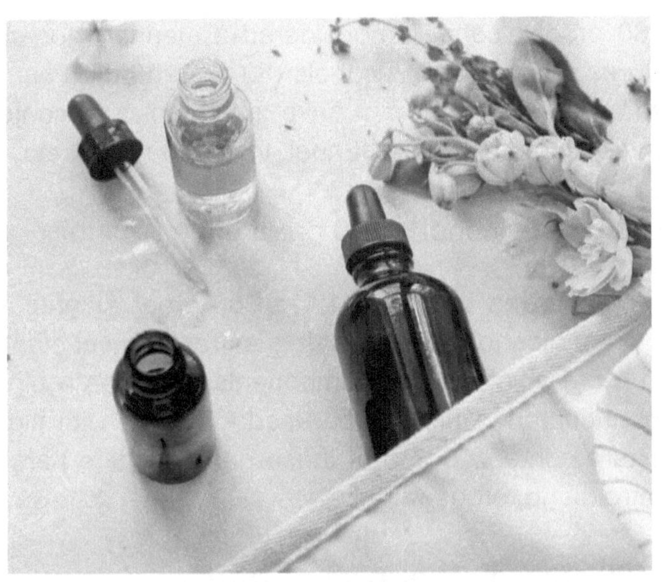

Ingredients Required For Tinctures

It is extremely easy to make tinctures at home, using the herb of your choice. Tinctures, as effective as they are, can be made in no time. You probably cannot tell for sure whether the tinctures are original or not if you are purchasing them from a nearby herbal store. It is always better to make them in your kitchen. Here is a general list of items that you will need to make tinctures at home.

- Alcohol
- 80 proof alcohol

80 proof alcohol is considered a standard for most tinctures. This type of Alcohols (80 proof Vodka) can be used on herbs that do not have much moisture content. Some of these herbs are fennel, thyme, bay, dill, etc.

- 80 proof alcohol + 190 proof grain alcohol

A mixture in the ratio (1:1) of 80 proof Alcohol and 190 proof alcohol can be used to extract the substances from more volatile plant components as it has a higher alcohol content. This can be used for herbs with higher moisture content. Some of these herbs include parsley, cilantro, sage, oregano, etc.

- 190 proof grain alcohol

190 proof grain alcohol is generally used for dissolving thick plant portions such as resins and gums. These are found in the dried plant matters like the bark of trees, etc. While it makes tinctures, which are strong in taste, it can also extract essential aromatics and oils in plants. It can somehow dehydrate the tincture, which might affect the long-term quality of the tincture.

Alternative To Alcohol

If you do not have access to alcohol or due to some other constraints, you are unable to utilize alcohol, you can alternatively use fire cider vinegar or food-grade glycerin. The difference is that it will then be called an extract instead of a tincture. This is an alternate method but serves the same function.

Herbs

Tinctures can be made with both, fresh and dried herbs. You can even use leaves, flowers, and berries to do the same. It is always best to use fresh herbs for tinctures as it will last longer and may also have considerable long-term effects.

No doubt, fresh herbs serves best for tinctures but are not readily available everywhere. Dried herbs are easiest to get your hands on because they last longer and do not rot easily.

Some of the most common herbs used for tincture these days are:

- Nettle
- Echinacea
- Licorice
- Elderberries
- Ashwagandha

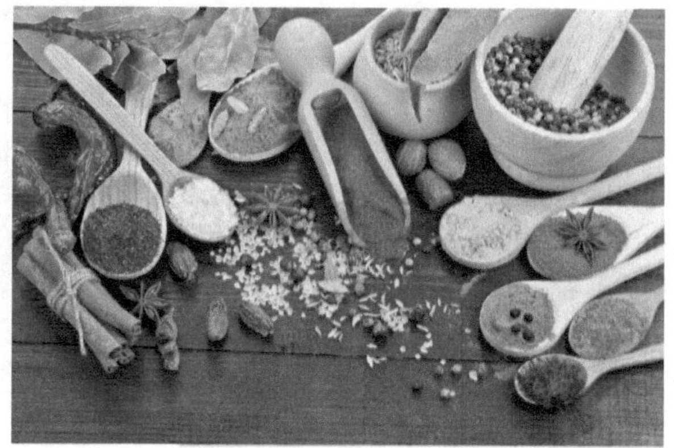

Instructions to make Tinctures

Step 01

Take a pint-sized glass jar with a lid. You will also use a piece of parchment or a plastic wrap. So, if you are using a jar with a metal lid than grab that piece of plastic too. Find a corner of a room in which this container can rest without much disturbance.

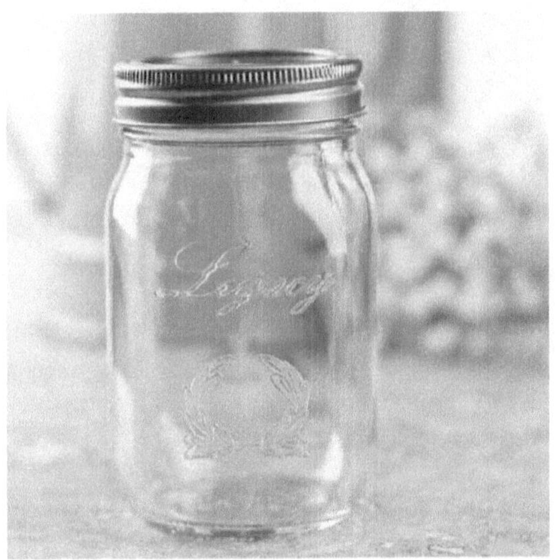

Step 02

Take a pestle or a mortar and finely chop your herbs. You have to chop them fine enough to fit the glass jar. Chopping the herbs gives them a considerable surface area to dissolve the liquid, that you will add later.

You can also toss the herbs directly into the jar without chopping them but then the strength of the tincture will be compromised.

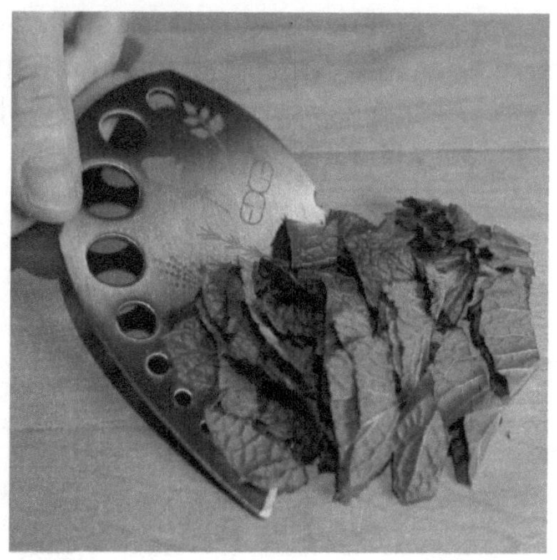

Step 03

Once you are done with Step 02, filled the rest of the jar with Alcohol. Remember to fill the jar because anything popping out above the liquid will start to mold. Make sure that the levels of liquid are an inch higher than your herbs. So, to keep the herbs from molding, submerge them well below the liquid surface.

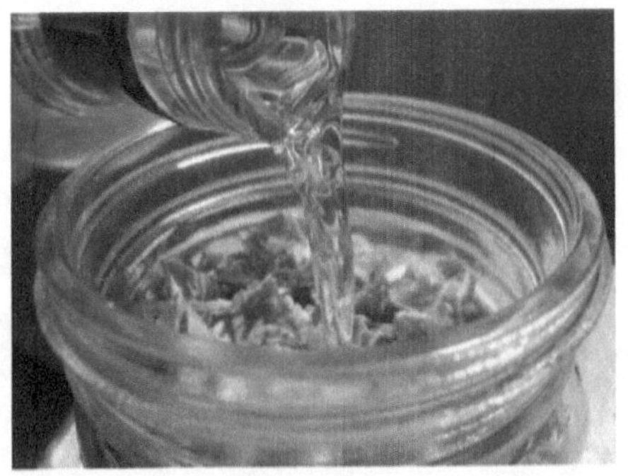

Step 04

Screw on the lid tightly. If you are using a jar with a metal lid, then you will have to wrap the mouth of the jar with a piece of plastic wrap. After wrapping the piece over the mouth, screw the lid and place the jar in a cabinet. Remember to keep the jar in a dry, cool, and dark place so that the extraction process could readily start.

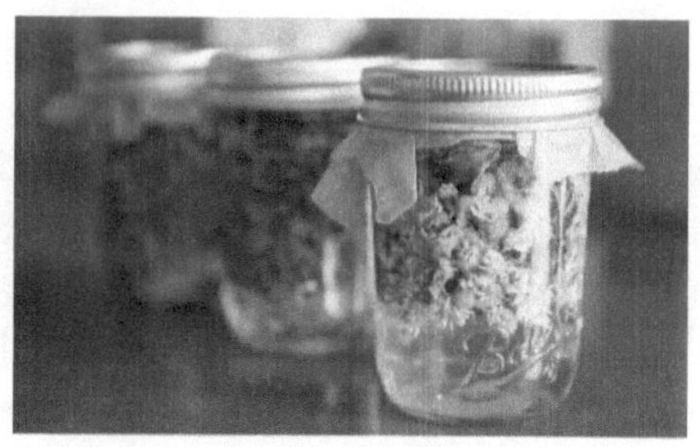

Step 05

Check on the jar every couple of days. Shake the jar now and then so that the herbs might alter their positions to make the extraction process more effective. Also, check to see if the alcohol hasn't evaporated too much. If you feel that the herbs are not submerged, then top it off with the same alcohol. Keep on checking the jar regularly for almost 8 weeks.

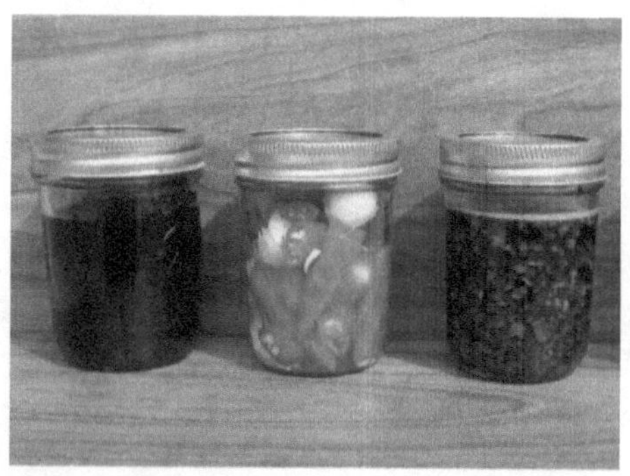

Step 06

After the extraction process is complete, take an amber dropper bottle. Remember to take the bottle with a fine-mesh strainer. Put the funnel in the amber bottle and pour all the liquid from the jar into the funnel. This will strain out all the herbs. To extract the remaining part of the tincture, take a cheesecloth and wrap the remaining herbs in the cloth. Squeeze the cheesecloth to extract the remains thoroughly.

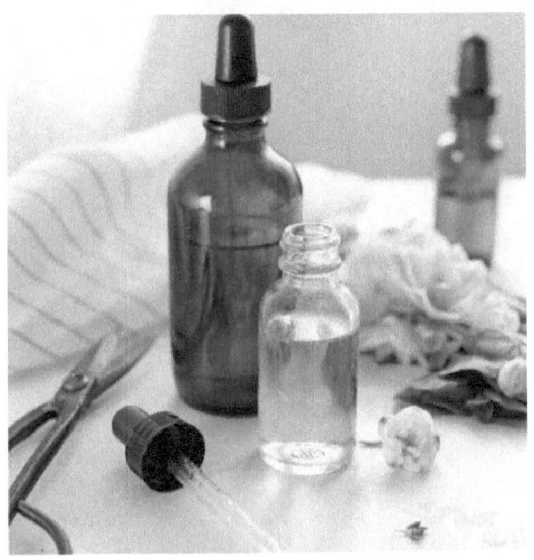

Step 07

If you have made more than one tinctures, then be sure you label them properly. When labeling the bottle write

- Herbs used

- Percent and Type of Alcohol
- Date and Time

This is it; you are ready with your tincture. You can make a tincture using the herbs of your liking. The advantages of each herb are explained in the previous chapters.

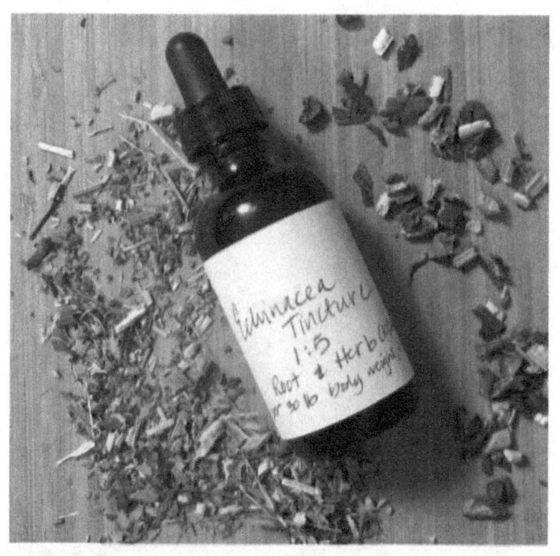

How To Use The Tincture

To utilize this tincture, you can use different methods.

1. You can always place a few drops directly under your tongue.
2. You can always add a few drops to a glass of water or a cup of tea.

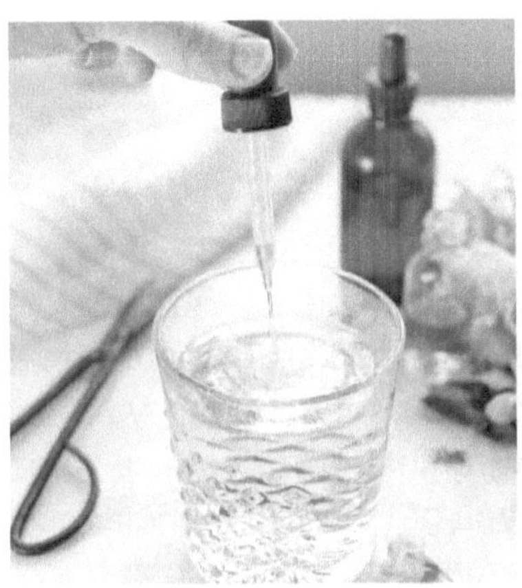

The amount of the tincture you are adding to the tea or water always depends on the strength of the tincture. It also depends on the herbs used because some herbs are stronger than others. Your body chemistry also influences the amount of tincture you might want to use. Most people like it light but some prefer it strong.

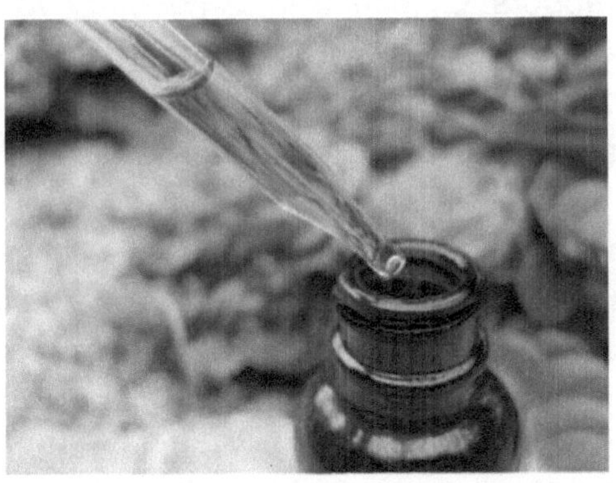

Chapter 6
Grow Your Own

There's always this pleasant, calming feeling about a person interacting with nature on a personal level. It is difficult to understand why not more people engage in growing their own produce when it's so easy and fun; plus, you get to save money once your little creations have matured and you can harvest them. So let's try growing those herbs right now!

Here's what you'll need to do:

Deciding Where to Grow

You'll have to figure out which is more preferable to you; either growing indoors (using containers) or growing outdoors. Objects that can destroy your plants or tamper with steady growth are strong enforcers here. The problem could be the dog outside or the kid inside; it's important to know which place is safest and will be most kind to your plant.

It's best to keep in mind that some herbs will have a harder time growing in containers because their root systems require ample space; herbs like horseradish, fennel, and lovage are some of these herbs while many others can grow perfectly fine in containers; those are like mint, chives, sage, bay, horehound, and winter savory. Knowing this, a container might be a great start for your seedling to mature, but some herbs might need to be plotted on prepared earth to grow well eventually.

Deciding Method of Growing

1. From Seeds

Acquiring seeds of the specific herb you require from a store or a mature plant and appending an environment to it that will stimulate the germination of the seed is required here. Various seeds of herbs have different needs and gestation periods and so acquiring information about this before proceeding with propagation is crucial or the seed could fail to germinate. Generally, most seeds of herbs germinate in temperatures approximated to 21°C with sufficient moisture supply and can take from a week to four weeks before they sprout seedlings.

(Tip: *Placing the seeds inside a closed plastic bag and misting the innards with water can ensure that there is sufficient humidity needed for germination of the seeds.*)

2. From Seedlings

If fortunate enough to already have seedlings of a herb, then preparations for propagation can begin immediately by placing the seedlings in plotted spaces on prepared earth.

3.   From Stem cuttings

It is possible to grow a herb by cutting part of the stem of a mature plant and placing it in water. Eventually, the stem cutting will grow roots and you'll be able to place it in the soil for further propagation.

Of course, it would be miraculous if every cutting of a certain herb could continue to propagate and so increasing optimal conditions (acquiring cuttings when herbs are going through fresh growth like after harvesting or during the spring here there is increased growth of foliage) is crucial for higher success rates

Preparing the Environment for Growth Before Propagation

1.   Area for Growth

You can grow your herbs in any pot-shaped vessels that can support them until when they reach maturity or you can prepare the land for growing by secluding a selected area and plotting the spacing between your herbs with the knowledge of the size of the plants once they reach maturity to avoid congestion. The typical spacing of the plants would be 10 inches to 16 inches apart which should ensure enough air and light to penetrate broad spaces of the plants.

2.   Equipment to Acquire

a.   For Indoor Growth

- Water-soluble fertilizer; organic matter is most suitable.
- Fluorescent grow lights that provide full-spectrum light at around 40 wattages to be placed above the growing plant.
- A watering can for irrigation or you can be creative and create an automated system that can irrigate your plants for you.
- A pesticide that can help control pest infestation.
- A cutting instrument for harvesting.
- Gardening gloves for protection from thorns and splinters.
- A hand trowel for placing seedlings.

b. For Outdoor Growth

- An irrigation system to supply the plants with water. This could be a person on a schedule with a watering can who can walk around to water the plants or an automated machine that can supply water on command or from following a schedule.
- A pesticide that can help control pest infestation.
- A rake to remove stones and other clogs.
- A spade to remove weeds or to add material to the soil such as fertilizer.
- A hand trowel for placing seedlings in the ground or for sowing.
- Gardening gloves for protection from thorns and splinters and other unwanted particles.

- A wheelbarrow to move gardening material around.

Conditions to Maintain While Advancing Towards Maturity

- Soil

  The seedlings require garden soil which is usually loam soil with various sized minerals of clay, silt, and sand; proportioned with more silt and clay than the sand; and contains a lot of organic matter which serves as nutrients and give it a workable texture.

- Fertilizer

  Herbs generally do not require heavy fertilizing as this can make the plant leaves and stems grow broad which would cause a lower concentration of the chemicals which the herb is being grown for so it is best to stick to organic matter and other light fertilizers alone as a source of nutrients for the plants if potency is of greater importance than quantity. This makes regular garden soil mixed with some organic fertilizer perfect for outdoor cultivation. Organic fertilizer is recommended to be added to the soil in liquid format
(soluble fertilizer in water) every two weeks, very sparingly when growing in pots.

- Light

  If it has been decided to grow the herbs indoors, then grow lights with full-spectrum
lights thrusting both warm and cool lights which mimic solar radiation should be placed above the plants. The

maturing seedlings should be kept under the light for up to around 14 hours which should mimic daylight exposure. Placing the plants close to a window where enough sunlight can seep through to cover the plant is also possible, but a minimum of six hours of sunlight exposure a day is required for most herbs to undergo enough photosynthesis to survive. Some herbs might require less light exposure than others, for example; mint, rosemary, and thyme can thrive under significantly low light and so it is best to see how to better expose the plants to daylight with minimal power wastage. If it has been decided to grow the herbs outside, there should be no obstruction from sunlight towards the plant.

- Irrigation

Watering the plant two to three times a week should be sufficient. The best way to water indoors is to allow the pots to dry out slightly in between waterings. To manage this well, place a finger inside the pot and it should be dry at about two inches deep. When this is so, then it is best to start watering again. The pot usually starts to dry from the top and so there should still be moisture below the pot with a good watering schedule being followed. This is done to encourage a healthy root system.

(Tip: Do not overwater the soil or the nutrients in it will be washed away more readily.)

(Tip: Do not water too quickly or the water will run through the soil without it absorbing enough of it.)

- Humidity

Hefty airflow all around the plant should be maintained as the air will supply the plant with humidity which should help keep moisture content high as the plant can lose moisture through transpiration when the air is dry at higher rates. Placing the plant under a fan or by a window while indoors can help with the proper circulation of air around the plant.
Regular misting of the plant with water should help slow the rate at which plants transpire.

- Drainage

Herbs grown in pots should have holes beneath them which should allow for the soil to dry out as certain herbs like bay, marjoram, oregano, thyme require to have soil that is left to dry slightly between the watering of the pots. Other herbs like rosemary should never have soil allowed to dry off completely and so it is important to have information on which drainage system is best for the type of herb you are trying to grow as many tend to rot in excessively moist soil.

- Temperature

Growing herbs have to be kept at temperatures approximated to 21°C during the day and around 13°C during the night. Some herbs can survive temperatures hovering as low as

5°C while others like basil cannot survive under 10°C and so research should be done on which temperatures the herb you're going to be growing can tolerate.

- Pest Control

       If an insect infestation is suspected, then it is best, to begin with, the least toxic and least expensive methods of fertilizing which include covering the leaves of the herbs with a water-soap solution of little soap concentration. A 5/400 ratio of soap to water solution is recommended.

       The application should be done every week to a point where the pests are no longer a problem. If the leaves appear to be affected by the solution, then lessen the soap's concentration in the water to a higher degree. Washing of the plant's leaves should be done before any kind of human consumption once the plant has reached maturity and can be exploited.

       A stronger pesticide could work with trickier pests that are resistant to the water-soap solution, especially a pesticide that is known to target the specific pest you spotted.

Harvesting After Complete Gestation Into Maturity

       Harvesting of herbs should be done when the plants have reached a maturity where there is a maximum concentration of the compounds responsible for the flavor and aroma and other health benefits of the herb of interest.

With mature annual herbs, up to 70% of their foliage can be cut and the plant can continue to grow. With perennial herbs, it is safe to remove up to a third of their foliage and the plant will still be able to survive and grow more foliage.

(Tip: Harvest the herbs before flowers begin to appear as this can predict slowing in leaf growth in the future. Cutting away from flowers can help ameliorate the situation; this should promote more leaf growth.)

(Tip: Use sharp equipment to cut away at the foliage while harvesting the plant to avoid great damage of the plant's xylem tissue and phloem tissue which are responsible for transporting food compounds, mineral salts, and water from the soil and leaves to all parts of the plant.)

Storing After Harvesting

After harvesting, it's best to consider which method will allow your herbs to remain fresh for longer. How you intend to use the herbs in the first place should help pinpoint how you'll be proceeding here as well.

There are specific things to do for how you intend to store your plants or how you intend to use them.

1. Drying
      Drying can help increase the concentration of some organic chemicals you seek from the herbs as water will evaporate, though with some other chemicals you might be seeking; most oils will remain as oils evaporate significantly slowly. Knowing which chemicals you're after is important before proceeding with this method of preservation. Some methods such as air drying are better than others in terms of retaining organic chemical quantity. There are various methods of doing this.

a. Air Drying
      This is considered the traditional method of drying herbs. It involves placing an assortment of harvested herbs in a loose bunch and placing them in a thin, plastic container with holes with ample ventilation, then placing it out to allow drying in the sun. This method is very time-consuming as it can take up to a month or sometimes longer for the herbs to dry out completely.
Another way this could be done is by scattering the herbs on trays and placing them under the sun which is preferable to the former when dealing with leafy herbs.

b. Drying With Heat

This can involve using anything from microwaves to ovens to food dehydrators.

- Using Microwaves

This method is considered risky as there is a higher chance of the herb charring so it is important to set the microwave to supply lower wattages of power; an approximated 800-watt power supply is preferable and time frames can vary depending on moisture content and microwave build; and so, when drying, continuously heat the herb until it reaches a point where the herb is crumbly, but don't proceed further to avoid charring.

- Using Ovens or Food Dehydrators

This method is a lot more forgiving than using microwaves as there is less potential for charring in ovens and food dehydrators and the process can be more readily controlled overall. A temperature of around 80°C maintained for 2-5 hours can ensure drying to the point where the herbs crumble with crushing.
For food dehydrators, following the owner's manual guidelines should ensure higher chances of success.

2. Freezing

This is considered to be the easiest way of storing a herb after harvesting. There will be a change in appearance over time, but flavor content will be maintained.

It is also possible to puree the herbs with minimal water addition and then freeze the paste, then break the pieces of frozen paste and use them later; when needed.

Conclusion

As we've discovered in the contents of this book, herbal medicine is not only the best healing system that combines balance, knowledge from various disciplines in the attempt to heal the human body in the least aggressive and non-invasive way possible, but also a fun and exciting subject that can benefit you and your loved ones in many ways. The research that supports herbalism as a relevant and resourceful type of medicine, is abundant.

When looking at the way it all started, at the history of herbalism, we can conclude easily that herbal medicine was the base for the scientific medicine we know today in the western world. Going through time we see how the ancient physicians followed by the new ones, have all believed it to be of massive importance to do research and write about the plants and remedies derived from them. Each one of them added on top of the other's research to form the basis of a more comprehensive medical system that unfortunately has lost its value throughout time, not because of its ineffectiveness but because humans didn't know how to combine the experimental science with herbalist medicine. We looked at different and specific plants, the most common ones, usually the ones most of us see around daily, we recognized their importance and usefulness and showed some of their most recorded health benefits.

Next, we looked at plants that can be used in teas, and more specifically plants that are not just delicious in teas but also ones that by drinking them regularly can improve our overall health. We recognized which plants are better in teas, in what specific areas of the body they affect, as well as looking at the main ingredients in terms of vitamins and minerals that make up the plant. We also gave you some recipes to take away and try for yourself, hoping you will get inspired and come up with some new and original ones.
After looking at the most simple ways of using plants for health benefits, such as in teas, we looked at a slightly more difficult use of herbs: in tinctures. Seeing how tinctures use alcohol for better absorption of the plant in the organism, we realized how beneficial they can be especially when desiring immediate results. The recipes we looked at hold great value and we hope you will try some of them and come to the same realizations.

At the beginning of this book, we promised that herbal medicine works. It would have been misleading and deceitful to promise such things if the research wouldn't have been available in such massive quantities. People all over the world find it oftentimes more successful in curing diseases for good, at times even uncurable by western medicine. There have been reports of such results in many countries, however, these are the ones more difficult to believe. I know a woman who was struggling with recurrent brain cancer for many years until she started taking purely plant supplements daily, having the doctors surprised with the results of after just a few months. I understand these examples don't hold much scientific credibility, though I believe most of them to be true. The less incredible results however have much more proof, not only in the number of people deciding to practice herbalism but also in the number of the ones who continue to buy plant-based remedies in very large quantities all over the world. Testimonies of such people are all over the internet and even the medical professionals believe in their benefits and prescribe all sorts of plant-based medicines to their patients.

After thoroughly looking at this amazing practice that is herbalism, or alternative medicine, however, you prefer to call it, there is one thing I would very much want you to take away from all this information.

Whenever you or someone you care about is faced with a health issue, think about this: the human body is an interconnected organism that needs nurturing and understanding, not only fixing. It is our most precious belonging and deserves to be treated with care and respect. More often than not, the symptoms are the ones we look at and try to fix, but the problem usually lays deeper. Understanding the difference between treating and healing the body will give you the most important resource in deciding whether or not herbalism is the best answer to your health issues.

Using this process when making a decision, will lead you to not only adopt herbal medicine as your preferred type of medicine but also to come to a greater understanding and love for your body.

Resources

- Weltz, Klein, Menrad. (2018). Why people use herbal medicine: insights from a focus-group study in Germany. BMC Complementary Medicine and Therapies. https://bmccomplementmedtherapies.biomedcentral.com/articles/10.1186/s12906-018-2160-6#Sec8https://drwaynejonas.com/the-proven-power-of-alternative-medicine-and-its-ability-to-heal/

- Sullivan, T. (2018, May 6). Modern Medicine vs. Alternative Medicine: Different Levels of Evidence. Policy & Medicine. https://www.policymed.com/2011/08/modern-medicine-vs-alternative-medicine-different-levels-of-evidence.html

- Villegas, H. (2019, June 4). How Herbs Changed My Life and Health (Why You Should Learn How to Use Herbs Too!) — All Posts. Healing Harvest Homestead. https://www.healingharvesthomestead.com/home/2019/4/20/how-herbs-transformed-my-health-and-life-plus-why-you-should-learn-about-using-herbs-too

- Wikipedia contributors. (2020, May 27). History of herbalism. Wikipedia. https://en.wikipedia.org/wiki/History_of_herbalism

- A Brief History of Herbalism. (2007). Herbs: Friends of Physicians, Praise of Cooks. http://exhibits.hsl.virginia.edu/herbs/brief-history/

- A Pagan's Guide to Herbalism II What is Herbalism? A Brief History & it's Connection to Paganism. (2019, January 16). [Video]. YouTube. https://www.youtube.com/watch?v=YTZOG4T0I3k

- Ancestral Herbalism. (2019, September 25). [Video]. YouTube. https://www.youtube.com/watch?v=B5AT04pxibM

- First Wednesdays: History of Herbalism in America. (2015, January 27). [Video]. YouTube. https://www.youtube.com/watch?v=HHGnfn_IeQw

- The Origins of Herbalism with Sarah Wu. (2018, December 18). [Video]. YouTube. https://www.youtube.com/watch?v=cM6rBFKmwd8

- The History of Herbalism. (2017, July 19). [Video]. YouTube. https://www.youtube.com/watch?v=Yv41MKdb3I4